CUT THE FAT!

The New Diabetic Cookbook

◇ ◇ ◇ ◇ ◇

By the Editors of Time-Life Books

TIME®
LIFE
BOOKS

Alexandria, Virginia

TIME-LIFE BOOKS IS A DIVISION OF TIME LIFE INC.

TIME-LIFE CUSTOM PUBLISHING

VICE PRESIDENT and PUBLISHER	Terry Newell
Project Manager	Jennifer Pearce
Director of Sales	Neil Levin
Special Sales Manager	Liz Ziehl
Managing Editor	Donia Ann Steele
Production Manager	Carolyn Mills Bounds
Quality Assurance Manager	Miriam P. Newton

Cut the Fat! was produced by Rebus, Inc., New York, New York

Recipe analysis by Hill Nutrition Associates

Library of Congress Cataloging-in-Publication Data
Cut the fat! : the new diabetic cookbook / from the editors of Time-Life Books.
p. cm.
Includes index.
ISBN 0-7835-4797-8
1. Diabetes—Diet therapy—Recipes. 2. Low-fat diet—Recipes.
I. Time-Life Books.
RC662.C88 1996
641.5'6314—dc20   95-47567
                                                CIP

Cover: Chicken, Potato, and Carrot Stew, page 42
Cover photograph by Vincent Lee

Note: This book is not intended as a substitute for medical advice. Please consult your physician or a registered
dietitian to determine the dietary guidelines that are appropriate for your health needs.

CONTENTS

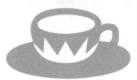

If you are one of the 14 million Americans living with diabetes, you've probably been asked, "Are you allowed to eat that?" Until recently, the answer most likely would have been, "No." This is because in the past, people with diabetes were subjected to a rigid, standardized diet. Now, there is good news: The American Diabetes Association has done away with this one-size-fits-all approach to meal planning and has approved more flexible guidelines, meeting the great variety of needs that exist.

The recipes in this cookbook are designed to provide a number of choices for people with diabetes, as well as for anyone who just wants to eat smarter. The complete nutrient and exchange breakdown of each recipe makes it easy to put together delicious meals that meet your own individual requirements.

The ingredients found in these recipes are available in most supermarkets, and the instructions are simple and easy to follow. In an effort to encourage healthful eating, the recipes derive no more than 30 percent of their calories from fat. (The nutrient breakdown for each recipe includes the percentage of calories that comes from fat.) And each dish is low in sodium, sugar, and cholesterol. Use this cookbook with confidence, as a guide to healthier cooking and eating habits for you and your family.

DIABETES

Commonly characterized by high blood sugar, the symptoms of

diabetes include increased thirst, frequent urination, increased hunger, fatigue, blurred vision, and unexplained weight loss. Type I (juvenile-onset) diabetes occurs primarily in children or young adults. People with Type I diabetes cannot produce their own insulin, a vital hormone produced in the pancreas that enables food to be converted into energy. Type I diabetes is treated with daily insulin injections that replace the insulin the body does not produce. Type II diabetes (adult-onset) usually occurs in people over age 40, and frequently those who develop it are overweight. This type of diabetes accounts for approximately 90 percent of all people who have diabetes and often goes undiagnosed. People with Type II diabetes usually produce some insulin, but it either is not enough or is not used efficiently by the body. In many cases, Type II diabetes may be treated solely through diet and exercise, but some people must take oral medication and/or insulin in addition.

NUTRITION COUNSELING

The latest nutrition guidelines from the American Diabetes Association focus on providing people with diabetes greater flexibility in meal planning by emphasizing the importance of an *individualized* diet, rather than assigning the same rigid diet to each person. They recommend that people with diabetes work with a registered dietitian to develop a meal plan tailored to their specific needs. The dietitian will take into consideration the following factors:

- Medication: Do you take insulin injections or oral medication?

- Physical condition: Do you have any conditions other than diabetes, such as high blood pressure, kidney problems, or obesity?
- Personal factors: Are there any foods you especially like or dislike? Do your religious beliefs affect your diet?
- Activity level: How often and when do you exercise?

DIETARY GOALS

The goal of nutrition counseling for people with diabetes is to improve overall health through optimal nutrition. This often means making changes in eating and exercise habits in order to improve blood sugar control.

The specific dietary goals of people with diabetes begin with the content of foods. The amount of carbohydrate, protein, and fat in foods will play a part in what, how much, and how often you eat. Some of the most important dietary elements in meal planning are:

Calories: The daily amount must be planned and adhered to in order to achieve or maintain a desired weight.

Carbohydrate: Will vary in amount depending on the person's individual needs and the recommendations of the healthcare provider.

Protein: Should account for 10 to 20 percent of the total daily calories. This represents less meat and fewer dairy products than most Americans normally consume.

Fat: The recommended percentage of calories from fat should be 30 percent or less but will vary according to the individual.

The different types of fat are monounsaturated (found in canola oil, olive oil, nuts, avocado), polyunsaturated (found in corn oil, safflower oil, sunflower oil, cottonseed oil), and saturated (found in meats, dairy products, coconut oil, palm oil, shortening).

It is best to limit saturated fats and choose foods containing more monounsaturated or polyunsaturated fat.

Sodium: Intake recommendations are the same as for the general population, with a range of 2,400 to 3,000 milligrams per day. (Range will differ for those with hypertension.)

Cholesterol: Daily intake should not exceed 300 milligrams.

Sugar: Can be used in the diet as long as it is counted as part of the total daily allowance of carbohydrate. This is also true of other sweeteners such as corn syrup, fruit juice, honey, sorbitol, and mannitol. Concentrated sweets usually contain little nutritive value and are often high in fat.

Non-Nutritive Sweeteners: Products such as aspartame, saccharin, and acesulfame are considered safe for people with diabetes and contain no nutritive value.

FOOD LABELS

Learning to read labels is an essential part of diabetes management. Any food with more than one ingredient must offer complete ingredient listings. Food labels provide values for calories, total fat, cholesterol, sodium, total carbohydrate, and protein. For all foods, it is important to check the serving size listed, because the portion size may not match the portion size of an exchange. Remember that whenever you choose new foods, you should monitor your blood sugar to see how the new food affects it.

EXCHANGE LISTS

The use of "exchanges" allows people with diabetes to follow a meal plan under varying conditions. It allows one food to be substituted for another. For example, within the carbohydrate group, you can exchange a starch for a fruit because they contain the same amount of carbohydrate per serving. In this cookbook, exchange values per serving are listed at the end of each recipe.

The chart below gives some rough values for a single exchange within the various food groups. For example, one vegetable

NUTRIENT VALUES OF EXCHANGE LISTS

The American Diabetes Association recently revised its Exchange Lists for Meal Planning to include the following groupings and nutrient content of exchanges.

Groups/Lists	Carbohydrate (grams)	Protein (grams)	Fat (grams)	Calories
Carbohydrate Group				
Starch	15	3	1 or less	80
Fruit	15	—	—	60
Milk				
Skim	12	8	0-3	90
Low-Fat	12	8	5	120
Whole	12	8	8	150
Other carbohydrates	15	varies	varies	varies
Vegetables	5	2	—	25
Meat and Meat Substitute Group				
Very Lean	—	7	0-1	35
Lean	—	7	3	55
Medium-Fat	—	7	5	75
High-Fat	—	7	8	100
Fat Group	—	—	5	45

exchange represents five grams of carbohydrate, two grams of protein, and 25 calories. A dietitian can help you determine the number of daily exchanges in the different food groups that is right for you.

For instance, Diabetic A might be advised to follow a daily meal plan of 1,200 calories consisting of roughly 150 grams of carbohydrate, 60 grams of protein, and 40 grams of fat. One possible combination of exchanges could result in a daily meal plan of 4 starches, 4 fruits, 2 skim milks, 2 vegetables, 4 lean meats, and 4 fats. For Diabetic B, with different health needs, the number of daily calories might be 2,000 with approximately 250 grams of carbohydrate, 100 grams of protein, and 66 grams of fat. For this person, a daily meal plan could consist of 8 starches, 5 fruits, 2 skim milks, 6 vegetables, 7 lean meats, and 8 fats.

The exchange lists are an essential part of diabetic meal planning. A full and detailed listing of exchanges can be obtained through your local branch of the American Diabetes Association, your dietitian, or by writing to or calling

> ADA Fulfillment Department
> P.O. Box 930850
> Atlanta, GA 31193-0850
> 1-800-232-6733

❖   ❖   ❖

For a person with diabetes, the ultimate goal of meal planning is to balance food intake with insulin in an effort to prevent the long-term complications of diabetes. The recipes in this cookbook can help you achieve that goal by adding variety and interest to your meals. Enjoy!

Gloria A. Elfert

Gloria A. Elfert, M.S., R.D./L.D.
The Johns Hopkins Diabetes Center

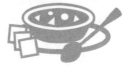

Vegetable Soup

2 teaspoons olive oil
1½ cups chopped onion
1 cup diced red bell pepper
⅔ cup diced celery
½ cup diced carrot
2 garlic cloves, minced
⅔ cup broccoli florets
⅓ cup thinly sliced zucchini
⅓ cup thinly sliced yellow squash
⅓ cup yellow cornmeal
¼ cup thinly sliced scallions
2 tablespoons grated Parmesan cheese

1 In a large saucepan, heat the oil over medium heat. Add the onion, bell pepper, celery, carrot, and garlic, reduce the heat to low, and cook about 10 minutes, or until the onions are soft.

2 Increase the heat to high and add 6 cups of water. Bring the soup to a boil and add the broccoli, zucchini, and yellow squash. Reduce the heat to medium-low and simmer about 7 minutes, or until the broccoli is tender.

3 Increase the heat to high and bring the soup to a rolling boil. Slowly pour in the cornmeal, whisking constantly. Continue whisking about 1 minute, or until the soup thickens. Remove the pan from the heat and ladle the soup into 4 bowls. Sprinkle each serving with scallions and Parmesan.

Serves 4

PER SERVING
EXCHANGES: ½ STARCH, 2½ VEGETABLES, ½ FAT
NUTRIENTS: 3G FAT/21%, 0.8G SATURATED FAT,
126 CALORIES, 2MG CHOLESTEROL, 78MG SODIUM,
21G CARBOHYDRATE, 4G PROTEIN, 4G DIETARY FIBER

Leek and Potato Soup

4 to 5 leeks (about 1 pound)
2 potatoes, peeled and quartered
1 cup thinly sliced celery
4 cups low-sodium chicken stock
2 cups skim milk
1 tablespoon chopped fresh parsley (optional)
White pepper

1 Cut off the root ends and green tops from the leeks. Halve the leeks lengthwise, separate the layers, and wash them thoroughly. Cut the leeks into 1-inch pieces.

2 In a large saucepan, combine the leeks, potatoes, celery, and stock. Bring to a boil, skimming off any scum. Reduce the heat and simmer, uncovered, about 40 minutes, or until the vegetables are tender. Cool the soup briefly, then purée in a blender or food processor or mash to a coarse purée by hand.

3 Return the soup to the saucepan, add the milk, and reheat the soup just until heated through; do not boil. Ladle the soup into 4 bowls or mugs and sprinkle with parsley (if using) and pepper.

Serves 4

PER SERVING
EXCHANGES: 1 STARCH, ½ SKIM MILK, 2 VEGETABLES
NUTRIENTS: 3G FAT/16%, 1G SATURATED FAT,
170 CALORIES, 2MG CHOLESTEROL, 220MG SODIUM,
31G CARBOHYDRATE, 10G PROTEIN, 2G DIETARY FIBER

Spiced Pumpkin Soup

2 teaspoons butter

¾ cup coarsely chopped onion

1 teaspoon curry powder

½ teaspoon ground cumin

2 cups canned or cooked pumpkin

¼ cup chopped fresh cilantro (optional)

2 teaspoons brown sugar

2 tablespoons tomato paste

¼ teaspoon black pepper

Pinch of salt

1   Melt the butter in a medium-size saucepan over medium heat. Add the onion and sauté 3 to 4 minutes, or until light golden. Add the curry powder and cumin, and cook, stirring, 1 minute.

2   Add the pumpkin, cilantro (if using), sugar, tomato paste, pepper, salt, and 3 cups of water, and stir gently to mix well. Bring the mixture to a boil, then cover the pan, reduce the heat to low, and simmer the soup about 30 minutes, or until the flavors are well blended.

Serves 4

PER SERVING

Exchanges: ½ starch, ¼ other carbohydrate, 1 vegetable, ½ fat
Nutrients: 2g fat/20%, 1.4g saturated fat, 88 calories, 5mg cholesterol, 126mg sodium, 17g carbohydrate, 2g protein, 3g dietary fiber

Chickpea and Escarole Soup

2 tablespoons olive oil

1 cup chopped onion

1 tablespoon minced garlic

½ teaspoon dried thyme

½ teaspoon dried oregano

8 cups coarsely chopped escarole leaves

2½ cups canned chickpeas, rinsed and drained

¼ cup long-grain white rice

1 cup frozen or canned corn kernels

2 tablespoons tomato paste

2 tablespoons lemon juice

1½ teaspoons salt

¼ teaspoon hot pepper sauce

Black pepper

1   In a 6- to 8-quart pot, heat the oil over medium heat. Stir in the onion, garlic, thyme, and oregano, and sauté 3 to 5 minutes, or until the onion is wilted. Add the escarole, chickpeas, and rice, and stir to coat lightly with oil. Add 10 cups of water, cover the pot, and bring to a boil. Reduce the heat and simmer, covered, 30 minutes.

2   Stir in the corn, tomato paste, and lemon juice. Return the soup to a boil, then cover the pan, reduce the heat, and simmer 30 minutes.

3   Add the salt and hot pepper sauce, and pepper to taste, and serve.

Serves 8

PER SERVING

Exchanges: 1¼ starches, ¾ vegetable, 1 fat
Nutrients: 5g fat/29%, 0.6g saturated fat, 154 calories, 0mg cholesterol, 563mg sodium, 23g carbohydrate, 5g protein, 5g dietary fiber

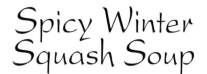

Spicy Winter Squash Soup

One 2½-pound acorn squash

One 12-ounce can spicy vegetable juice

1 cup chopped green bell pepper

1 cup fresh or frozen corn kernels

1 tablespoon chopped fresh basil,
   or 1 teaspoon dried basil

Pinch of salt

1 Preheat the oven to 400°.

2 Line a medium-size baking pan with foil.

3 Halve the squash, remove the seeds, and place the squash cut side down in the pan. Bake 40 minutes, or until the squash is tender when pierced with a knife. Set aside to cool about 15 minutes.

4 Scoop the squash into a large saucepan and mash it with a potato masher or fork to remove any large lumps (or purée the squash in a food processor or blender). Add 1½ cups of water, the vegetable juice, bell pepper, corn, basil, and salt, and bring to a boil over medium-high heat. Reduce the heat to low and simmer 10 to 15 minutes. Serve hot, or cool the soup to room temperature and then refrigerate it and serve it chilled.

Serves 6

PER SERVING
EXCHANGES: 1¼ STARCHES, ½ VEGETABLE
NUTRIENTS: 0.5G FAT/5%, 0.1G SATURATED FAT,
96 CALORIES, 0MG CHOLESTEROL, 204MG SODIUM,
24G CARBOHYDRATE, 2G PROTEIN, 6G DIETARY FIBER

Puréed Carrot Soup

1 tablespoon corn oil
1 cup coarsely chopped onion
½ cup chopped shallots
3 cups low-sodium chicken stock
2 cups thinly sliced carrots
2 cups drained canned sliced beets
4 thin lemon slices for garnish (optional)
Four 2-ounce multigrain rolls

1 Heat the oil in a medium-size saucepan over medium heat. Add the onion and shallots and cook, stirring frequently, 10 minutes. Add the stock and carrots, increase the heat to medium-high, and bring the mixture to a boil. Cover the pan, reduce the heat to medium-low, and simmer 15 minutes, or until the carrots are tender. Add the beets and cook for 5 minutes longer.

2 Remove the pan from the heat and allow the soup to cool slightly. Using a slotted spoon, transfer the solids to a food processor, and process 1 minute, or until puréed.

3 Return the purée to the pan. Let the soup cool, then cover and refrigerate it until well chilled. Stir the soup to reblend it, then ladle it into 4 bowls and garnish with lemon slices (if using). Warm the rolls in the oven briefly and serve with the soup.

Serves 4

PER SERVING
EXCHANGES: 2 STARCHES, 3¾ VEGETABLES, 1 FAT
NUTRIENTS: 8G FAT/27%, 1.5G SATURATED FAT,
270 CALORIES, 0MG CHOLESTEROL, 586MG SODIUM,
46G CARBOHYDRATE, 10G PROTEIN, 8G DIETARY FIBER

Spinach-Mushroom Soup

2 garlic cloves, thinly sliced
2 teaspoons butter or margarine
¾ pound fresh spinach, washed and cut into
    ¼-inch-wide strips
4 cups low-sodium chicken stock
2 cups sliced fresh mushrooms, or ⅔ cup
    rinsed and drained canned mushrooms
¼ teaspoon black pepper
Pinch of salt
Four 2-ounce whole-wheat rolls

1 Sauté the garlic in the butter in a large saucepan over low heat 2 to 3 minutes.

2 Add the spinach, stock, mushrooms, pepper, and salt, and bring to a boil. Cover the pan, reduce the heat to low, and simmer the mixture 8 to 10 minutes, or until the vegetables are tender. Serve the soup with the rolls.

Serves 4

PER SERVING
EXCHANGES: 2 STARCHES, 1¼ VEGETABLES, 1 FAT
NUTRIENTS: 7G FAT/30%, 2.6G SATURATED FAT,
211 CALORIES, 5MG CHOLESTEROL, 535MG SODIUM,
33G CARBOHYDRATE, 12G PROTEIN, 7G DIETARY FIBER

Cream of Tomato Soup with Croutons

One 14-ounce can plum tomatoes,
    with their liquid
1 cup tomato juice
½ pound small red potatoes, peeled and diced
1¼ cups diced red bell pepper
1 cup coarsely chopped onion
2 tablespoons chopped fresh
    cilantro or parsley (optional)
1 garlic clove, peeled and crushed
¼ teaspoon black pepper
1 slice whole-wheat bread
¾ cup skim milk

1 Preheat the oven to 375°.

2 In a medium-size saucepan, combine the tomatoes and their liquid, tomato juice, potatoes, bell pepper, onion, cilantro (if using), garlic, and black pepper and bring to a boil over medium heat. Cover the pan, reduce the heat to low, and simmer 15 minutes.

3 To make the croutons, cut the bread into ½-inch cubes, spread them on a baking sheet, and bake 5 to 10 minutes, or until golden; set aside to cool.

4 Remove the pan of soup from the heat and set aside to cool for a few minutes. Purée the soup in a food processor or blender 1 minute, or until smooth. With the machine running, gradually add the milk.

5 Return the soup to the pan and reheat it over medium-high heat; do not boil. Ladle the soup into bowls and top with croutons. *Serves 4*

PER SERVING
EXCHANGES: ¾ STARCH, ¼ SKIM MILK, 2½ VEGETABLES
NUTRIENTS: 1G FAT/7%, 0.2G SATURATED FAT,
135 CALORIES, 1MG CHOLESTEROL, 450MG SODIUM,
28G CARBOHYDRATE, 5G PROTEIN, 4G DIETARY FIBER

Black-Eyed Pea Soup

2 tablespoons plus 2 teaspoons margarine
1 cup chopped onion
2 garlic cloves, chopped
One 10-ounce package frozen black-eyed peas,
    thawed
One 14-ounce can plum tomatoes,
    with their liquid
1 cup diced carrots
1 cup diced celery
1 cup frozen lima beans
½ cup low-sodium chicken stock
1 teaspoon ground cumin
1 teaspoon coriander seeds (optional)
¼ teaspoon black pepper

1 Melt the margarine in a large saucepan over medium-high heat. Add the onion and garlic and sauté 2 to 3 minutes, or until the onion begins to turn translucent. Add the black-eyed peas, the tomatoes with their liquid, the carrots, celery, lima beans, stock, cumin, coriander seeds (if using), pepper, and 1 cup of water, and stir to combine. Bring the mixture to a boil, then cover the pan, reduce the heat to low, and simmer 30 minutes.

2 Using a slotted spoon, transfer about two-thirds of the solids from the soup to a food processor or blender and purée.

3 Return the purée to the saucepan and stir to combine. Bring the soup to a boil over medium-high heat and simmer it, stirring constantly, 2 minutes, or until heated through. Ladle the soup into 4 bowls and serve. *Serves 4*

PER SERVING
EXCHANGES: 1¾ STARCHES, 2½ VEGETABLES, 1¾ FATS
NUTRIENTS: 9G FAT/30%, 2G SATURATED FAT,
267 CALORIES, 0MG CHOLESTEROL, 331MG SODIUM,
38G CARBOHYDRATE, 12G PROTEIN, 9G DIETARY FIBER

Creamy Mushroom Barley Soup

½ pound onions

2 garlic cloves

2 cups low-sodium chicken stock

6 tablespoons barley

½ pound fresh mushrooms, or 1 cup rinsed and
drained canned mushrooms

¼ cup chopped fresh parsley (optional)

2 tablespoons chopped fresh dill,
or 2 teaspoons dried dill

1　Peel and coarsely chop the onions and garlic; set aside.

2　Bring the stock and 2 cups of water to a boil in a medium-size saucepan over medium-high heat. Stir in the onions, garlic, and barley, cover the pan, reduce the heat to low, and simmer 45 minutes.

3　Meanwhile, wash, trim, and coarsely chop the mushrooms; set aside.

4　Add the mushrooms to the soup, cover the pan, and simmer another 15 minutes.

5　Using a slotted spoon, transfer the solids to a food processor or blender and process until puréed.

6　Return the purée to the saucepan, then stir in the parsley (if using) and the dill. Bring the soup to a boil over medium-high heat, then ladle it into 4 bowls.

Serves 4

PER SERVING

EXCHANGES: ¾ STARCH, 1¾ VEGETABLES, ½ FAT
NUTRIENTS: 2G FAT/16%, 0.5G SATURATED FAT,
110 CALORIES, 0MG CHOLESTEROL, 65MG SODIUM,
21G CARBOHYDRATE, 6G PROTEIN, 5G DIETARY FIBER

Tomato-Rice Soup

2 pounds fresh, ripe tomatoes, or one
32-ounce can tomatoes, with their liquid

1½ cups cooked brown rice (¾ cup raw)

1 cup chopped celery

½ cup chopped onion

¼ cup chopped fresh basil, or 1 tablespoon
dried basil

3 tablespoons tomato paste

2 garlic cloves, chopped

Pinch of salt

¼ teaspoon black pepper

1 bay leaf

1　If using fresh tomatoes, core and quarter them. Place the tomatoes in a large nonreactive pot and add ½ cup of the rice, the celery, onion, basil, tomato paste, garlic, salt, pepper, bay leaf, and 1 quart of water. Bring the mixture to a boil over medium heat, then cover the pot, reduce the heat to low, and simmer the soup about 30 minutes, stirring occasionally and breaking up the tomatoes with the edge of the spoon.

2　Remove the pot from the heat, uncover it, and allow the soup to cool about 30 minutes; remove and discard the bay leaf.

3　Transfer the soup to a food processor or blender, in 2 batches if necessary, and process until puréed.

4　Return the soup to the pot and stir in the remaining rice. Reheat the soup over medium heat. Divide it among 6 bowls and serve.

Serves 6

PER SERVING

EXCHANGES: ¾ STARCH, 2 VEGETABLES, ¼ FAT
NUTRIENTS: 1G FAT/8%, 0.2G SATURATED FAT,
108 CALORIES, 0MG CHOLESTEROL, 120MG SODIUM,
23G CARBOHYDRATE, 3G PROTEIN, 3G DIETARY FIBER

White Bean and Corn Soup

2 strips bacon, diced
¾ cup coarsely diced red bell pepper
½ cup chopped carrots
½ cup diced onions
2 garlic cloves, minced
1½ tablespoons unbleached all-purpose flour
1 cup skim milk
1 bay leaf
½ teaspoon salt
¼ teaspoon white pepper
¼ teaspoon dried sage
1½ cups canned white beans, rinsed and
    drained
1 cup frozen or canned corn kernels

1   In a medium-size saucepan over medium-low heat, cook the bacon about 6 minutes, or until crisp; pour off and discard all but 1 tablespoon of fat.

2   Add the bell pepper, carrots, onions, and garlic to the saucepan and cook, covered, about 7 minutes, or until the vegetables are softened.

3   Add the flour and cook, stirring, 1 minute. Add 1 cup of water, the milk, bay leaf, salt, pepper, and sage and cook another 4 minutes, or until the soup is slightly thickened. Add the beans and cook another 10 minutes, or until the flavors are well blended.

4   Add the corn and cook just until heated through. Remove and discard the bay leaf.   *Serves 4*

PER SERVING
EXCHANGES: 1½ STARCHES, ¼ SKIM MILK, 1 VEGETABLE, 1 FAT
NUTRIENTS: 5G FAT/23%, 1.5G SATURATED FAT, 198 CALORIES, 6MG CHOLESTEROL, 574MG SODIUM, 30G CARBOHYDRATE, 10G PROTEIN, 5G DIETARY FIBER

Chicken Soup with Carrots, Potatoes, and Spinach

1 small chicken (about 2 pounds), skinned, all
    visible fat removed
1 onion, peeled
1 celery stalk
8 to 12 parsley sprigs
1 bay leaf
1 teaspoon ground cumin
1 sprig fresh thyme,
    or ¼ teaspoon dried thyme
1 whole bulb of garlic, outer papery coating
    removed, the bulb cut in half crosswise
½ teaspoon salt
1 pound boiling potatoes, peeled and sliced
1 pound carrots, sliced ¼-inch thick
4 ounces fresh spinach, washed, stemmed,
    and sliced into ½-inch-wide strips

1   Put the chicken into a large pot and add 6 cups of water. Bring the water to a boil, then reduce the heat and simmer the chicken for 10 minutes, frequently skimming off the foam that rises to the surface. Add the onion, celery, parsley, bay leaf, cumin, thyme, garlic, and salt, and simmer 45 minutes, or until the chicken is tender.

2   Place a colander over a large bowl and pour the contents of the pot into it. Leave the chicken to cool in the colander.

3   Return the broth to the pot and bring it to a boil. Add the potatoes, reduce the heat, and cover the pot; then simmer 10 minutes, or until the potatoes are just tender. Remove the potatoes with a slotted spoon and set them aside.

4   Add the carrots to the simmering broth, cover the pot, and continue to cook 15 to 20 minutes, or until the carrots are very tender.

5   Meanwhile, remove the meat from the chicken and cut or tear it into bite-size pieces. Reserve the meat; discard the bones and the remaining solids in the colander.

6   When the carrots are cooked, purée half of them

with half of the broth in a food processor or blender. Transfer the contents to a bowl; then purée the remaining carrots and broth. Pour all the liquid back into the pot. Add the potatoes, chicken, and spinach leaves. Reheat the soup gently before serving.

Serves 4

PER SERVING
EXCHANGES: 1 STARCH, 3 VEGETABLES, 3 VERY LEAN MEATS, ¾ FAT
NUTRIENTS: 4G FAT/13%, 0.9G SATURATED FAT, 274 CALORIES, 76MG CHOLESTEROL, 425MG SODIUM, 32G CARBOHYDRATE, 27G PROTEIN, 6G DIETARY FIBER

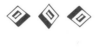

Cauliflower-Cheese Soup

2 teaspoons butter
1 cup chopped leeks
2 cups reduced-sodium chicken stock
1 large sweet potato (about 14 ounces), peeled and cut into ½-inch-thick slices
4 cups cauliflower florets
1 tablespoon coarse-grain mustard
2 tablespoons chopped fresh parsley (optional)
⅓ cup reduced-fat Swiss cheese, grated

1   Melt the butter in a medium-size pan over medium heat. Add the leeks and sauté 3 to 5 minutes, or until tender. Add the stock and 1 cup of water and bring to a boil. Add the sweet potato and cauliflower; reduce the heat to low, cover the pan, and simmer about 20 minutes, or until the potato is tender.

2   Remove the pan from the heat and allow the soup to cool slightly. Transfer the soup to a food processor or blender (working in batches, if necessary) and process it for 1 to 2 minutes, or until puréed, scraping down the sides of the container with a spatula.

3   Add the mustard and parsley (if using), and stir until combined. Ladle the soup into 4 bowls and top each serving with grated cheese.

Serves 4

PER SERVING
EXCHANGES: 1 STARCH, 2½ VEGETABLES, ¼ LEAN MEAT, 1 FAT
NUTRIENTS: 5G FAT/26%, 2.5G SATURATED FAT, 174 CALORIES, 10MG CHOLESTEROL, 160MG SODIUM, 27G CARBOHYDRATE, 8G PROTEIN, 5G DIETARY FIBER

Lentil Minestrone

1 teaspoon olive oil
2 cups coarsely diced green bell pepper
1½ cups coarsely chopped onions
1 cup diced celery
2 ounces lean ground chuck
2 garlic cloves, minced
⅓ cup dried lentils
¼ cup white rice
4 small tomatoes, cut into 1-inch cubes
2 ounces elbow macaroni (½ cup)
1 tablespoon lime juice
¾ teaspoon salt
½ teaspoon dried oregano
¼ teaspoon black pepper
¼ cup grated Parmesan cheese

1   Heat the oil in a Dutch oven or large heavy-gauge saucepan over medium heat. Add the bell pepper, onions, celery, ground chuck, and garlic, and cook, stirring, about 5 minutes, or until the vegetables are softened. Stir in the lentils, rice, tomatoes, macaroni, and 2 quarts of water, cover the pan, and bring to a boil. Reduce the heat and simmer 45 minutes.

2   Add the lime juice, salt, oregano, and black pepper. Sprinkle with the Parmesan before serving.

Serves 4

PER SERVING
EXCHANGES: 2 STARCHES, 3 VEGETABLES, ½ LEAN MEAT, ¾ FAT
NUTRIENTS: 5G FAT/17%, 1.8G SATURATED FAT, 272 CALORIES, 13MG CHOLESTEROL, 557MG SODIUM, 44G CARBOHYDRATE, 14G PROTEIN, 6G DIETARY FIBER

Black Bean Soup

1½ cups orange juice

1¼ cups canned black beans, rinsed and
   drained

2 carrots, cut into 3-inch pieces

1 cup finely chopped onion

1 teaspoon ground cumin

4 orange slices, for garnish (optional)

1 Place the juice, beans, carrots, onion, and cumin
in a medium-size nonreactive saucepan. Bring to a
boil, reduce the heat to low, and simmer, covered, 20
minutes. Set the soup aside to cool briefly, then
process it in a food processor or blender until just
puréed.

2 Reheat the soup over low heat, then ladle it into
4 bowls and garnish with orange slices (if using).

Serves 4

PER SERVING

EXCHANGES: ½ STARCH, ¾ FRUIT, 1¼ VEGETABLES
NUTRIENTS: 1G FAT/7%, 0G SATURATED FAT,
130 CALORIES, 0MG CHOLESTEROL, 178MG SODIUM,
27G CARBOHYDRATE, 5G PROTEIN, 5G DIETARY FIBER

Italian Split Pea Stew

1 tablespoon butter

1½ cups chopped onion

1 garlic clove, minced

One 35-ounce can plum tomatoes, with their
   liquid

1 cup dried yellow split peas

¾ teaspoon dried oregano

1 bay leaf

1 Melt the butter in a medium-size saucepan over
medium heat. Add the onions and garlic and sauté 10
minutes, or until golden. Add the tomatoes and their
liquid, the split peas, oregano, bay leaf, and 1 cup of

water and bring to a boil. Reduce the heat to medium-
low, cover the pan, and simmer the stew 25 minutes, or
until the split peas are tender.

2 Remove and discard the bay leaf. Ladle the stew
into 4 bowls and serve.

Serves 4

PER SERVING

EXCHANGES: 2 STARCHES, 3 VEGETABLES, ¾ FAT
NUTRIENTS: 4G FAT/13%, 2G SATURATED FAT,
269 CALORIES, 8MG CHOLESTEROL, 443MG SODIUM,
46G CARBOHYDRATE, 15G PROTEIN, 6G DIETARY FIBER

Herbed Gazpacho

Two 14½-ounce cans peeled tomatoes, with
   their liquid

1½ cups finely chopped unpeeled cucumber

½ cup finely chopped scallions

⅓ cup finely diced celery

¼ cup chopped fresh basil, or 1 tablespoon
   plus 1 teaspoon dried basil

2 tablespoons red wine vinegar

1 small garlic clove, minced

½ teaspoon black pepper

Pinch of salt

1 In a large bowl combine the tomatoes and their
liquid, cucumber, scallions, celery, basil, vinegar, garlic,
pepper, and salt; stir well to break up the tomatoes.
Cover the bowl and refrigerate the gazpacho 4 hours,
or until thoroughly chilled.

2 Stir the soup to reblend it before serving.

Serves 4

PER SERVING

EXCHANGES: 2½ VEGETABLES
NUTRIENTS: 0.6G FAT/9%, 0.1G SATURATED FAT,
58 CALORIES, 0MG CHOLESTEROL, 380MG SODIUM,
13G CARBOHYDRATE, 3G PROTEIN, 3G DIETARY FIBER

Onion Soup with Shallot Toasts

4 cups coarsely chopped leeks
2 cups low-sodium chicken stock
1 cup coarsely chopped onion
2 garlic cloves, chopped
2 tablespoons sherry
½ teaspoon dried thyme
1 bay leaf
⅛ teaspoon white pepper
1 tablespoon butter or margarine
1 cup coarsely chopped shallots
6 ounces Italian bread, cut into 4 slices
2 tablespoons grated Parmesan cheese

1 In a medium-size saucepan combine the leeks, stock, onion, garlic, sherry, thyme, bay leaf, white pepper, and 1½ cups of water, and bring to a boil over medium-high heat. Cover, reduce the heat to low, and simmer 1 hour.

2 Remove and discard the bay leaf. Using a slotted spoon, transfer the solids from the soup to a food processor or blender and process until puréed. Return the purée to the pan, cover, and set aside.

3 Preheat the broiler.

4 Meanwhile, melt the margarine in a small skillet over medium-high heat. Add the shallots and sauté 1 to 2 minutes, or until they begin to brown.

5 Toast the bread slices under the broiler 1 minute on each side, or until golden; set aside.

6 Reheat the soup over medium-high heat, stirring occasionally, 3 to 5 minutes, or until heated through.

7 Meanwhile, divide the shallots among the slices of toast, sprinkle them with Parmesan, and broil for another minute, or until golden brown and fragrant. Divide the soup among 4 bowls, top with the toasts, and serve.

Serves 4

PER SERVING
EXCHANGES: 1½ STARCHES, 5 VEGETABLES, 1¼ FATS
NUTRIENTS: 7G FAT/23%, 3G SATURATED FAT, 279 CALORIES, 10MG CHOLESTEROL, 409MG SODIUM, 49G CARBOHYDRATE, 10G PROTEIN, 4G DIETARY FIBER

Corn Chowder

1 tablespoon olive oil
½ cup chopped scallions
2 tablespoons flour
2½ cups reduced-sodium chicken stock
10 ounces peeled and diced red potatoes
2 cups frozen corn kernels, thawed
½ cup diced red bell pepper
1 teaspoon dried thyme
¼ teaspoon black pepper
1 cup lowfat (1%) milk

1 In a medium saucepan over medium-high heat, warm the oil until hot but not smoking. Add the scallions and cook, stirring, 1 to 2 minutes, or until softened. Add the flour and cook, stirring until the flour is no longer visible, 10 to 20 seconds.

2 Add the stock and potatoes, cover the pan, and bring to a boil. Reduce the heat to low and simmer for 10 minutes, or until the potatoes are tender.

3 Using a slotted spoon, transfer about half the potatoes to a shallow bowl; lightly mash them with a fork.

4 Return the mashed potatoes to the pan. Add the corn, bell pepper, thyme, and black pepper, and return to a boil over medium-high heat. When the chowder comes to a boil, add the milk and cook, stirring gently, for about 1 minute.

Serves 4

PER SERVING
EXCHANGES: 2 STARCHES, ¼ LOWFAT MILK, ½ VEGETABLE, 1 FAT
NUTRIENTS: 5G FAT/21%, 0.9G SATURATED FAT, 219 CALORIES, 2MG CHOLESTEROL, 444MG SODIUM, 38G CARBOHYDRATE, 9G PROTEIN, 4G DIETARY FIBER

Noodle Soup with Vegetables

2 tablespoons olive oil
2½ cups diced carrots
1½ cups chopped scallions
1 green bell pepper, seeded and diced
3 cups low-sodium chicken stock
6 ounces linguine
⅓ cup chopped fresh parsley (optional)
2 tablespoons chopped fresh dill,
   or 2 teaspoons dried
½ teaspoon salt
½ teaspoon black pepper

1 Heat the oil in a medium-size skillet over medium heat. Add the carrots, scallions, and bell pepper, and sauté 4 minutes, or until the carrots are softened. Add the stock and 1 cup of water and bring the mixture to a simmer.

2 Break the linguine into 2-inch lengths and stir it into the soup.

3 When the soup returns to a simmer, stir in the parsley (if using), dill, salt, and black pepper, and cook another 10 minutes, or until the linguine is al dente. Ladle the soup into 6 bowls and serve. *Serves 6*

PER SERVING
EXCHANGES: 1½ STARCHES, 1½ VEGETABLES, 1¼ FATS
NUTRIENTS: 6G FAT/28%, 1G SATURATED FAT,
190 CALORIES, 0MG CHOLESTEROL, 263MG SODIUM,
30G CARBOHYDRATE, 6G PROTEIN, 3G DIETARY FIBER

Fresh Tomato Soup

2 large tomatoes (1 pound total weight),
   cored and quartered
5 garlic cloves, chopped
4 tablespoons chopped fresh basil
2 tablespoons grated Parmesan cheese
1 tablespoon butter or margarine
1 large all-purpose potato, peeled and
   coarsely diced
1 cup thickly sliced carrots
¾ cup coarsely chopped scallions
1 cup low-sodium chicken stock
1 cup canned red kidney beans, rinsed
   and drained
1 cup fresh or frozen green peas
½ teaspoon salt

1 Place the tomatoes, garlic, 3 tablespoons of the basil, and Parmesan in a food processor or blender, and process until just blended, scraping down the sides of the container with a rubber spatula.

2 Melt the butter in a medium-size saucepan over medium-high heat. Add the potato, carrots, and scallions, and sauté 3 to 4 minutes, or until the scallions are limp. Add the tomato mixture, stock, kidney beans, and ½ cup of water and bring to a boil. Cover the pan, reduce the heat to low, and simmer 20 to 25 minutes, or until the potato is tender.

3 Add the remaining 1 tablespoon basil, the peas, and salt, and cook another 5 minutes. *Serves 8*

PER SERVING
EXCHANGES: ¾ STARCH, 1¼ VEGETABLES, ½ FAT
NUTRIENTS: 3G FAT/26%, 1.3G SATURATED FAT,
103 CALORIES, 5MG CHOLESTEROL, 246MG SODIUM,
16G CARBOHYDRATE, 5G PROTEIN, 4G DIETARY FIBER

Bean and Smoked Turkey Salad

¼ cup low-sodium chicken stock
2 tablespoons Dijon mustard
2 tablespoons lemon juice
1 tablespoon plus 1 teaspoon olive oil
1 garlic clove, minced
Black pepper
3 tablespoons finely chopped fresh basil,
    or 1 tablespoon dried basil
1 large head romaine lettuce, torn into bite-
    size pieces
3½ cups frozen baby lima beans, thawed
3 cups fresh pineapple chunks
1 medium-size red onion, thinly sliced
6 plum tomatoes, cut into wedges
2 cups seedless grapes
2 ounces smoked turkey, cut into strips
12 whole toasted almonds

1   In a small bowl combine the stock, mustard, lemon juice, oil, and garlic. Add pepper to taste and whisk until smooth. Stir in the basil; set aside.

2   Place the romaine in a large serving bowl. Add the lima beans, pineapple, onion, tomatoes, grapes, and turkey, and toss gently to combine. Add the dressing and toss again. Cover and refrigerate 3 hours, or until the salad is well chilled and the flavors are blended.

3   Divide the salad among 6 plates and scatter the almonds on top.

Serves 6

PER SERVING
EXCHANGES: 1¾ STARCHES, 1¼ FRUITS, 1½ VEGETABLES, ½ LEAN MEAT, 1 FAT
NUTRIENTS: 6G FAT/18%, 0.8G SATURATED FAT, 299 CALORIES, 5MG CHOLESTEROL, 289MG SODIUM, 52G CARBOHYDRATE, 13G PROTEIN, 9G DIETARY FIBER

Black Bean Salad

⅓ cup white wine vinegar
1 tablespoon corn oil
1 tablespoon Dijon mustard
1 teaspoon dark sesame oil
1 garlic clove, peeled and minced
1 teaspoon dried tarragon
¼ teaspoon salt
¼ teaspoon black pepper
2 cups canned black beans, rinsed and drained
1 cup diced celery
1 red bell pepper, thinly sliced
2 cups sliced carrots
1 cup canned sliced beets, drained
2 cups shredded romaine lettuce

1   In a large bowl whisk together the vinegar, corn oil, mustard, sesame oil, garlic, tarragon, salt, and black pepper. Add the beans, celery, and bell pepper, and toss well; set aside at room temperature.

2   Bring 2 cups of water to a boil in a medium-size saucepan over medium-high heat. Add the carrots and cook 5 minutes, or until crisp-tender. Drain the carrots, cool under cold running water, and set aside to drain.

3   Cut the beets into matchstick strips. Add the beets, carrots, and romaine to the salad, and toss to combine. Let the salad stand at room temperature at least 1 hour before serving.

Serves 6

PER SERVING
EXCHANGES: ¾ STARCH, 1½ VEGETABLES, ¾ FAT
NUTRIENTS: 4G FAT/29%, 0.4G SATURATED FAT, 126 CALORIES, 0MG CHOLESTEROL, 422MG SODIUM, 18G CARBOHYDRATE, 5G PROTEIN, 5G DIETARY FIBER

Red Bean and Rice Salad

2 tablespoons vegetable oil

1 cup brown rice

2½ cups low-sodium chicken stock

1 cup canned red kidney beans, rinsed and drained

¼ cup sliced celery

¼ cup chopped onion

¼ cup chopped green bell pepper

¼ cup chopped red bell pepper

1 tablespoon chopped fresh parsley (optional)

1 tablespoon red wine vinegar

½ teaspoon hot pepper sauce

2 cups shredded lettuce

1 Heat 1 tablespoon of the oil in a medium-size saucepan over medium-high heat. Add the rice and sauté until lightly browned. Add the stock and bring to a boil. Reduce the heat and simmer the rice, covered, 50 minutes, or until the rice is tender and the broth is completely absorbed. Drain the rice in a colander and set aside to cool at least 30 minutes.

2 When cool, transfer the rice to a bowl. Add the remaining oil and the other remaining ingredients except the lettuce, and toss until well combined. Cover and refrigerate 2 hours.

3 To serve, line a platter with shredded lettuce and mound the salad on top.

Serves 4

PER SERVING

EXCHANGES: 2¾ STARCHES, 1¼ VEGETABLES, 2 FATS
NUTRIENTS: 10G FAT/29%, 1.7G SATURATED FAT, 310 CALORIES, 0MG CHOLESTEROL, 188MG SODIUM, 48G CARBOHYDRATE, 10G PROTEIN, 5G DIETARY FIBER

Herbed Pinto Bean Salad

2 tablespoons low-sodium chicken stock

2 tablespoons white wine vinegar

1 garlic clove, minced

2 tablespoons chopped fresh parsley (optional)

1½ teaspoons chopped fresh basil, or ½ teaspoon dried basil

1 teaspoon dried tarragon

¼ teaspoon salt

¼ teaspoon black pepper

3 cups canned pinto beans, rinsed and drained

1 For the dressing, in a small bowl whisk together the stock, vinegar, garlic, parsley (if using), basil, tarragon, salt, and pepper.

2 Place the beans in a medium bowl and pour the dressing over them. Cover the bowl and refrigerate at least 3 hours, or overnight, to allow the flavors to blend.

Serves 2

PER SERVING

EXCHANGES: 3 STARCHES, 1¼ VERY LEAN MEATS, ½ FAT
NUTRIENTS: 2G FAT/7%, 0.3G SATURATED FAT, 277 CALORIES, 0MG CHOLESTEROL, 1,058MG SODIUM, 46G CARBOHYDRATE, 18G PROTEIN, 13G DIETARY FIBER

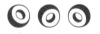

Black-Eyed Pea and Lentil Salad

½ cup dried lentils
¼ teaspoon plus ⅛ teaspoon salt
One 10-ounce package frozen black-eyed peas, thawed
½ cup finely chopped onion
¼ cup chopped fresh parsley (optional)
1½ teaspoons lemon juice
1 teaspoon Dijon mustard
1 garlic clove, minced
½ teaspoon dried thyme
⅛ teaspoon black pepper
1 teaspoon olive oil
2 tablespoons low-sodium chicken stock

1 Place the lentils in a medium-size saucepan with cold water to cover by 1 inch. Bring to a boil over medium heat and stir in ¼ teaspoon of the salt; cover, reduce the heat to low, and simmer 20 minutes, or until the lentils are tender, adding more water if necessary.

2 About 5 minutes before the lentils are done, add the black-eyed peas to the saucepan to heat through.

3 Drain the lentils and peas and transfer them to a medium-size bowl. Stir in the onion and parsley (if using).

4 For the dressing, in a small bowl whisk together the lemon juice, mustard, garlic, thyme, pepper, and the remaining ⅛ teaspoon salt. Slowly whisk in the oil, then add the stock, whisking constantly. Pour the dressing over the peas and lentils and toss well.

Serves 6

PER SERVING
EXCHANGES: 1½ STARCHES, ¾ VERY LEAN MEAT, ¼ FAT
NUTRIENTS: 1G FAT/7%, 0.2G SATURATED FAT,
133 CALORIES, 0MG CHOLESTEROL, 166MG SODIUM,
22G CARBOHYDRATE, 9G PROTEIN, 4G DIETARY FIBER

Potato, Cucumber, and Bell Pepper Salad

1 pound small red potatoes
1 small cucumber
1 red bell pepper
2 garlic cloves, peeled
1 cup lowfat buttermilk
2 tablespoons lowfat sour cream
2 tablespoons coarsely chopped red onion
½ teaspoon salt
¼ teaspoon pepper
1 tablespoon chopped fresh parsley (optional)

1 Bring a large pot of water to a boil. Scrub the potatoes, cut them into 1-inch cubes, and boil them about 15 minutes, or until tender.

2 Meanwhile, peel, seed, and dice the cucumber. Seed the bell pepper and cut it into 1-inch squares. Bring a medium-size saucepan of water to a boil. Blanch the cucumber 1 minute; remove with a slotted spoon and cool under cold water. Blanch the bell pepper in the same water 2 minutes; remove and cool under cold water. Blanch the garlic 4 minutes; drain and set aside.

3 Drain the potatoes and set aside to cool slightly. For the dressing, place ⅓ cup of potatoes and ⅓ cup of buttermilk in a food processor or blender; add the garlic and process until puréed. Stir in the sour cream and remaining buttermilk.

4 In a large bowl combine the remaining potatoes, cucumber, bell pepper, and onion. Add the dressing, salt, and pepper, and toss gently to combine. Sprinkle the salad with parsley (if using) and serve.

Serves 4

PER SERVING
EXCHANGES: 1¼ STARCHES, ¼ LOWFAT MILK, 1 VEGETABLE
NUTRIENTS: 2G FAT/12%, 1G SATURATED FAT,
146 CALORIES, 6MG CHOLESTEROL, 324MG SODIUM,
28G CARBOHYDRATE, 5G PROTEIN, 3G DIETARY FIBER

Spicy Potato and Chickpea Salad

1 tablespoon olive oil
½ cup chopped onion
2 garlic cloves, chopped
2 tablespoons white wine
3 tablespoons low-sodium chicken stock
2 tablespoons red wine vinegar
¼ teaspoon salt
1 teaspoon ground cumin
¼ teaspoon paprika
⅛ teaspoon ground cloves
Pinch of ground red pepper
⅔ cup canned chickpeas, rinsed and drained
4 medium-size potatoes, boiled and cut into
    1-inch pieces
½ cup bottled sliced roasted red peppers
    or pimientos
4 pitted black olives, halved
¼ cup chopped scallions
1½ tablespoons chopped fresh parsley
    (optional)

1 In a medium-size skillet, heat the oil until hot but not smoking. Add the onion and garlic and cook 1 minute, tossing to coat with oil, then cover and cook 4 to 5 minutes, or until the onion is soft.

2 Add the wine and boil gently until almost all of the liquid has evaporated. Add the stock, vinegar, salt, cumin, paprika, cloves, and ground red pepper, and simmer another 2 minutes.

3 Remove the skillet from the heat, add the chickpeas and potatoes, and toss gently. Add the pepper strips, olives, scallions, and parsley (if using), and toss again. Serve the salad at room temperature.

Serves 4

PER SERVING

EXCHANGES: 2 STARCHES, ½ VEGETABLE, 1 FAT
NUTRIENTS: 5G FAT/23%, 0.6G SATURATED FAT,
200 CALORIES, 0MG CHOLESTEROL, 273MG SODIUM,
35G CARBOHYDRATE, 5G PROTEIN, 4G DIETARY FIBER

Sweet Potato and Apple Salad

1½ pounds small sweet potatoes
¼ cup plain nonfat yogurt
3 tablespoons nonfat mayonnaise
1 tablespoon fresh lime juice
¾ teaspoon grated lime zest
¼ teaspoon salt
¼ teaspoon black pepper
1 large tart apple, unpeeled
2 stalks celery
⅓ cup chopped walnuts

1 Preheat the oven to 400°. Line a baking sheet with foil. Cut a few slits in each sweet potato as steam vents. Place the potatoes on the baking sheet and bake for 30 minutes, or until tender.

2 Meanwhile, in a large serving bowl, combine the yogurt, mayonnaise, lime juice, lime zest, salt, and pepper.

3 Coarsely chop the apple, add it to the dressing, and toss to coat. Add the celery and walnuts and stir to combine.

4 When the potatoes are cool enough to handle but still warm, peel them and cut them into bite-size pieces. Add the warm potatoes to the serving bowl and toss to coat with the dressing. Serve the salad at room temperature.

Serves 4

PER SERVING

EXCHANGES: 2¼ STARCHES, ½ FRUIT, 1¼ FATS
NUTRIENTS: 7G FAT/27%, 0.7G SATURATED FAT,
238 CALORIES, 0MG CHOLESTEROL, 259MG SODIUM,
42G CARBOHYDRATE, 4G PROTEIN, 5G DIETARY FIBER

Wild Rice Salad with Orange Dressing

1 cup wild rice

One 10-ounce package frozen Brussels
    sprouts, thawed

⅓ cup freshly squeezed orange juice

2 tablespoons vegetable oil

½ teaspoon pure orange extract

¼ teaspoon black pepper

Pinch of salt

1 cup slivered red bell pepper

2 tablespoons chopped fresh mint,
    or 2 teaspoons dried mint

4 large romaine lettuce leaves

1 Bring 3½ cups of water to a boil in a medium-size saucepan over medium-high heat. Add the rice, reduce the heat to low, and simmer, partially covered, for 45 minutes.

2 Cut the sprouts in half and set aside to drain on paper towels.

3 Remove the pan of rice from the heat and stir in the orange juice, oil, orange extract, black pepper, and salt. Stir in the Brussels sprouts, bell pepper, and mint. Let the mixture cool slightly, then transfer to a large bowl, cover with plastic wrap, and refrigerate overnight, stirring occasionally.

4 To serve, line a platter with the romaine and mound the salad on top.   *Serves 4*

PER SERVING

EXCHANGES: 2¼ STARCHES, 1¼ VEGETABLES, 1½ FATS
NUTRIENTS: 8G FAT/28%, 1G SATURATED FAT,
256 CALORIES, 0MG CHOLESTEROL, 46MG SODIUM,
40G CARBOHYDRATE, 9G PROTEIN, 5G DIETARY FIBER

Greek Salad

2 large cucumbers

½ cup plain lowfat yogurt

¼ cup chopped fresh mint, or 1 tablespoon
    plus 1 teaspoon dried mint

3 tablespoons lemon juice

4 plum tomatoes

4 ounces romaine lettuce, torn into bite-size
    pieces

¼ cup chopped scallions

1 ounce feta cheese, crumbled

1 Peel the cucumbers and halve them lengthwise. For the dressing, seed one cucumber half, cut it into large chunks, and process in a food processor or blender 15 to 20 seconds, or until puréed. Add the yogurt, mint, and lemon juice and process another 5 to 10 seconds, scraping down the sides of the container with a rubber spatula; set aside.

2 Cut the remaining cucumber halves lengthwise into quarters, then cut crosswise into ¼-inch-thick slices. Cut the tomatoes into large dice. Place the romaine, cucumber, tomatoes, and scallions in a large bowl and toss to combine. Sprinkle the feta over the salad and, just before serving, add the dressing and toss well.   *Serves 2*

PER SERVING

EXCHANGES: 2½ STARCHES, ½ LOWFAT MILK,
1½ VEGETABLES, ½ MEDIUM FAT MEAT
NUTRIENTS: 5G FAT/14%, 3G SATURATED FAT,
322 CALORIES, 16MG CHOLESTEROL, 231MG SODIUM,
52G CARBOHYDRATE, 21G PROTEIN, 10G DIETARY FIBER

Orzo Vegetable Salad

1½ cups orzo (rice-shaped pasta), or other
   small pasta shapes
¼ cup apple juice
3 tablespoons white wine vinegar
2 tablespoons plus 2 teaspoons vegetable oil
2 teaspoons Dijon mustard
½ teaspoon ground ginger
½ teaspoon black pepper
Pinch of salt
½ pound cherry tomatoes, halved
1 cup canned black beans, rinsed and drained
1 cup cooked green peas
1 large yellow bell pepper, diced

1   Bring a medium-size saucepan of water to a boil.
Add the orzo and cook 8 to 10 minutes, or according
to the package directions. Transfer the orzo to a
colander, cool under cold running water, and set aside
to drain.

2   In a medium-size bowl combine the apple juice,
vinegar, oil, mustard, ginger, pepper, and salt and stir
to combine. Add the tomatoes, beans, peas, bell pepper, and orzo and stir to combine. Serve the salad at
room temperature or chilled.   *Serves 6*

PER SERVING

EXCHANGES: 3 STARCHES, 1 VEGETABLE, 1½ FATS
NUTRIENTS: 7G FAT/20%, 0.9G SATURATED FAT,
312 CALORIES, 0MG CHOLESTEROL, 157MG SODIUM,
51G CARBOHYDRATE, 10G PROTEIN, 5G DIETARY FIBER

Apple, Celery, and Pasta Salad

5 ounces elbow macaroni (1¼ cups)
¼ cup red wine vinegar
1½ tablespoons olive oil
1 tablespoon frozen apple juice concentrate,
   thawed
¾ teaspoon oregano
½ teaspoon salt
¼ teaspoon black pepper
1 bunch celery
1 pound McIntosh apples, peeled, diced, and
   tossed with 2 tablespoons lemon juice
1½ cups frozen lima beans, cooked and drained
⅔ cup thinly sliced radishes
½ small head escarole or green-leaf lettuce,
   separated into leaves
1½ ounces Parmesan cheese

1   Bring a large saucepan of water to a boil. Add the
macaroni and cook 8 minutes, or according to the
package directions; drain, rinse under cold water, and
set aside to drain thoroughly.

2   For the dressing, whisk together the vinegar, oil,
apple juice concentrate, oregano, salt, and pepper;
set aside.

3   Trim and thinly slice the celery and add it to the
apples. Add the macaroni, lima beans, radishes, and
dressing and toss well.

4   Using a vegetable peeler or a sharp knife, cut the
Parmesan into thin shavings; set aside.

5   Line a platter with escarole or lettuce leaves and
mound the apple mixture on top. Scatter the Parmesan shavings over the salad and serve.   *Serves 4*

PER SERVING

EXCHANGES: 2½ STARCHES, 1 FRUIT, 1 VEGETABLE,
½ HIGH FAT MEAT, 1 FAT
NUTRIENTS: 10G FAT/24%, 2.9G SATURATED FAT,
371 CALORIES, 8MG CHOLESTEROL, 568MG SODIUM,
59G CARBOHYDRATE, 14G PROTEIN, 8G DIETARY FIBER

Tuna-Rice Salad

1 cup reduced-sodium chicken stock
1 cup water
1 cup rice
2 garlic cloves, minced
1 large yellow or green bell pepper
1 pint cherry tomatoes
4 scallions
½ cup chopped fresh dill, or 2 teaspoons dried
⅓ cup lemon juice
2 tablespoons olive or vegetable oil
1 tablespoon Dijon mustard
½ teaspoon black pepper
¼ teaspoon salt
1 can (6½ ounces) water-packed tuna, drained
1 small head Boston or iceberg lettuce,
    separated into leaves

1 In a medium saucepan, bring the chicken stock and water to a boil. Add the rice and garlic, reduce the heat to low, cover, and simmer 20 minutes, or until the rice is tender and all the liquid is absorbed. When the rice is done, remove it from the heat and turn it into a large bowl to cool slightly; fluff the rice with a fork or spoon to separate the grains and speed the cooling.

2 Meanwhile, cut the bell pepper into bite-size pieces. Halve the cherry tomatoes. Coarsely chop the scallions and dill.

3 To make the lemon-pepper dressing, in a small bowl, combine the lemon juice, olive oil, mustard, black pepper, and salt.

4 When the rice has cooled slightly, add the bell pepper, tomatoes, scallions, dill, tuna, and lemon-pepper dressing. Toss lightly to combine.

5 Serve the rice salad mounded on lettuce leaves.

Serves 6

PER SERVING
EXCHANGES: 1½ STARCHES, 1½ VEGETABLES, 1 VERY LEAN MEAT, 1 FAT
NUTRIENTS: 5G FAT/21%, 0.7G SATURATED FAT, 217 CALORIES, 12MG CHOLESTEROL, 340MG SODIUM, 30G CARBOHYDRATE, 12G PROTEIN, 1G DIETARY FIBER

Penne and Vegetable Salad

6 ounces fresh or ⅓ cup frozen asparagus,
    trimmed and cut into 1-inch pieces
¼ pound greens beans, trimmed and cut into
    1-inch pieces
2½ cups broccoli florets
6 cups coarsely chopped spinach
¼ pound penne pasta
1¼ cups coarsely chopped scallions
1 cup frozen peas, thawed
¾ cup coarsely diced red bell pepper
¼ cup red wine vinegar
2 tablespoons olive oil
½ teaspoon red pepper flakes, or to taste
½ teaspoon salt

1 Bring a large pot of water to a boil. Blanch the asparagus, green beans, and broccoli together in the boiling water 3 minutes. Reserving the boiling water, use a large slotted spoon (or a strainer) to transfer the blanched vegetables to a colander; cool under cold water, drain, and transfer to a large bowl.

2 Blanch the spinach 1 minute; drain in a colander, cool under cold water, and drain again. Add the blanched spinach to the bowl.

3 Refill the pot and bring the water to a boil. Cook the pasta according to package directions; drain, rinse well, and drain again.

4 Add the pasta to the bowl of blanched vegetables. Add the scallions, peas, bell pepper, vinegar, oil, red pepper flakes, and salt and toss well. Serve the salad at room temperature or chilled.

Serves 6

PER SERVING
EXCHANGES: 1 STARCH, 2½ VEGETABLES, 1 FAT
NUTRIENTS: 5G FAT/25%, 0.7G SATURATED FAT, 180 CALORIES, 0MG CHOLESTEROL, 273MG SODIUM, 27G CARBOHYDRATE, 9G PROTEIN, 6G DIETARY FIBER

Chicken-Cucumber Salad with Tarragon

½ cup chicken stock
1½ teaspoons dried tarragon
2 garlic cloves, minced
¼ teaspoon black pepper
¾ pound skinless, boneless chicken breast
    halves, thinly sliced
1 tablespoon olive oil
1 tablespoon white wine vinegar
⅓ cup plain lowfat yogurt
½ teaspoon salt
1 medium cucumber, peeled and cubed
1 large red bell pepper, coarsely chopped
8 Boston lettuce leaves

1 In a medium saucepan, bring the chicken stock, half of the tarragon, the garlic, and the black pepper to a boil over medium-high heat. Add the chicken slices and return to a boil. Reduce the heat to low, cover, and simmer, stirring occasionally, until the chicken is cooked through, about 7 minutes.

2 In a small bowl, combine the oil, vinegar, yogurt, salt, and remaining tarragon.

3 Transfer the chicken to a serving bowl (discard the stock). Add the cucumber, bell pepper, and yogurt dressing, and toss to combine.

4 Line individual serving plates with 2 lettuce leaves and spoon the salad on top.   *Serves 4*

PER SERVING

EXCHANGES: ¼ LOWFAT MILK, ½ VEGETABLE, 2½ VERY LEAN MEATS, ¾ FAT
NUTRIENTS: 5G FAT/28%, 0.9G SATURATED FAT, 159 CALORIES, 50MG CHOLESTEROL, 472MG SODIUM, 6G CARBOHYDRATE, 22G PROTEIN, 1G DIETARY FIBER

Beef and Barley Salad

½ cup pearl barley
2 cups low-sodium beef stock
1 pint cherry tomatoes
4 scallions
½ pound sliced lean roast beef
½ cup raisins
3 tablespoons lemon juice
2 tablespoons red wine or cider vinegar
2 tablespoons olive oil
2 tablespoons Dijon mustard
2 teaspoons grated lemon zest (optional)
½ teaspoon pepper

1 In a medium saucepan, combine the barley and beef stock, and bring to a boil over high heat. Reduce the heat to low, cover, and simmer until the barley is just tender, about 50 minutes.

2 Meanwhile, cut the cherry tomatoes into quarters. Coarsely chop the scallions. Cut the roast beef into thin strips.

3 In a serving bowl, combine the tomatoes, scallions, roast beef, and raisins.

4 In a small saucepan or skillet, combine the lemon juice, vinegar, oil, mustard, lemon zest (if using), and pepper. Cook over medium heat until just heated through, 3 to 4 minutes.

5 Pour the dressing over the vegetables and roast beef and toss to combine. Set aside until the barley is done.

6 Add the hot barley to the serving bowl and stir to combine. Serve the salad warm, at room temperature, or chilled.   *Serves 4*

PER SERVING

EXCHANGES: 1¼ STARCHES, 1 FRUIT, 1 VEGETABLE, 2 MEDIUM FAT MEATS, 1 FAT
NUTRIENTS: 11G FAT/29%, 2.4G SATURATED FAT, 344 CALORIES, 46MG CHOLESTEROL, 266MG SODIUM, 38G CARBOHYDRATE, 23G PROTEIN, 6G DIETARY FIBER

Layered Salad with Blue Cheese Dressing

2¼ ounces blue cheese, crumbled
½ cup plain lowfat yogurt
¼ cup nonfat sour cream
3 tablespoons chopped parsley
2 teaspoons Dijon mustard
2 teaspoons cider vinegar
¼ teaspoon black pepper
1 tablespoon chicken stock
¼ teaspoon garlic powder
2 ounces French bread, cubed
4 cups shredded romaine lettuce
2 cups grated carrots
24 cherry tomatoes
2 medium red bell peppers, slivered
1 hard-cooked egg, minced

1 Preheat the broiler.

2 To make the dressing, in a medium bowl combine the blue cheese, yogurt, sour cream, parsley, mustard, vinegar, and ⅛ teaspoon of the black pepper. Stir to combine.

3 To make the croutons, in a small bowl, combine the chicken stock, garlic powder, and remaining pepper. Add the bread cubes and toss to coat. Toast the seasoned bread cubes under the broiler for 1 to 2 minutes on each side or until evenly browned.

4 In a clear glass bowl, layer the salad as follows: half of the lettuce, all of the carrots, half of the tomatoes, the rest of the lettuce, all of the bell peppers, and the rest of the tomatoes. Sprinkle the minced egg and the croutons evenly over the top.

5 Just before serving, spoon the dressing evenly over the top of the salad.

Serves 8

PER SERVING
EXCHANGES: ¼ STARCH, 1¼ VEGETABLES, ½ HIGH FAT MEAT
NUTRIENTS: 3G FAT/27%, 1.8G SATURATED FAT, 100 CALORIES, 33MG CHOLESTEROL, 231MG SODIUM, 12G CARBOHYDRATE, 6G PROTEIN, 2G DIETARY FIBER

Italian Bread Salad

1 large ripe tomato
¼ cup tomato juice
3 tablespoons balsamic vinegar
2 teaspoons olive oil
¼ teaspoon dried thyme
Pinch each of salt and black pepper
2 bell peppers (preferably 1 red and 1 green), sliced and blanched in boiling water
5 ounces green beans, trimmed and blanched
2½ cups cubed whole-wheat bread

1 For the dressing, core and quarter the tomato, place it in a blender, and process until puréed. Add the tomato juice, vinegar, oil, thyme, salt, and black pepper and process until blended.

2 Place the blanched vegetables in a large bowl; add the bread cubes and the dressing and toss to combine. Cover the bowl and refrigerate for at least 2 hours, or until the bread has absorbed the dressing.

Serves 2

PER SERVING
EXCHANGES: 1½ STARCHES, 2½ VEGETABLES, 1½ FATS
NUTRIENTS: 7G FAT/30%, 1.1G SATURATED FAT, 211 CALORIES, 0MG CHOLESTEROL, 420MG SODIUM, 35G CARBOHYDRATE, 7G PROTEIN, 6G DIETARY FIBER

Three-Melon Salad

3 tablespoons white wine vinegar, or to taste
2 teaspoons safflower oil
1 tablespoon lemon juice
½ teaspoon salt
4 cups 1-inch cantaloupe chunks
3 cups 1-inch honeydew chunks
4 cups watermelon balls or chunks
2 ounces lowfat dry-curd cottage cheese or
    farmer cheese
½ cup chopped fresh mint leaves (optional)
4 large romaine lettuce leaves, washed and
    trimmed
2 tablespoons coarsely chopped pecans

1 For the dressing, in a small bowl, whisk together the vinegar, oil, lemon juice, and salt; set aside.

2 Combine the cantaloupe, honeydew, and watermelon in a large bowl, add the dressing, and toss gently. Cover the bowl and refrigerate at least 1 hour.

3 Just before serving, crumble the cheese into a small bowl, add the mint (if using), and mash with a fork to combine.

4 Line a serving platter with the romaine leaves and mound the melon on it. Sprinkle the cheese over the melon and scatter the pecans on top. *Serves 4*

PER SERVING
EXCHANGES: 2½ FRUITS, ¾ LEAN MEAT, 1 FAT
NUTRIENTS: 7G FAT/29%, 0.4G SATURATED FAT,
221 CALORIES, 5MG CHOLESTEROL, 351MG SODIUM,
39G CARBOHYDRATE, 6G PROTEIN, 4G DIETARY FIBER

Pear and Endive Salad

1 very ripe small pear (about 3 ounces), plus
    4 large pears (about 6 ounces each)
3 tablespoons lemon juice
3 tablespoons apple juice
1 tablespoon chopped fresh parsley (optional)
1 tablespoon nonfat sour cream
6 ounces Belgian endive, separated into leaves
1 ounce Gorgonzola cheese or other blue
    cheese

1 For the dressing, peel and core the small pear. Cut it into large chunks, place in a small bowl, and mash with a fork until smooth. Stir in 2 tablespoons of the lemon juice, the apple juice, parsley (if using), and sour cream; set aside.

2 Halve, stem, and core but do not peel the remaining pears. Cut the pears lengthwise into ¼-inch-thick slices, then place them in a medium-size bowl and toss with the remaining lemon juice.

3 Line a serving platter with the endive leaves and arrange the pear slices on top. Crumble the cheese over the pears and drizzle the dressing over the salad.
Serves 4

PER SERVING
EXCHANGES: 1½ FRUITS, ¼ VEGETABLE, ¼ HIGH FAT MEAT
NUTRIENTS: 3G FAT/23%, 1.5G SATURATED FAT,
115 CALORIES, 6MG CHOLESTEROL, 106MG SODIUM,
22G CARBOHYDRATE, 3G PROTEIN, 4G DIETARY FIBER

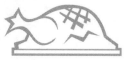

Oven-Baked Chicken Nuggets

2 garlic cloves, peeled
¼ cup parsley sprigs
4 slices stale bread
¼ cup grated Parmesan cheese
½ teaspoon onion powder
½ teaspoon black pepper
¼ teaspoon salt
1 tablespoon chilled butter or margarine
1 pound skinless, boneless chicken breasts
1 egg white

1   Preheat the oven to 425°. Line a baking sheet with foil and spray with nonstick cooking spray.

2   Place the garlic cloves and parsley in a food processor or blender. Process until finely chopped. Tear the bread into small pieces and add it to the parsley mixture, then add the Parmesan, onion powder, pepper, and salt, and process, pulsing the machine on and off, until the bread is coarse crumbs.

3   Cut the butter into small pieces and add it to the processor. Process until the butter is completely incorporated. Transfer the breading to a paper or plastic bag.

4   Cut the chicken into 1-inch cubes. In a medium-size bowl, beat the egg white. Add the chicken and stir to moisten well.

5   Drain the chicken cubes in a colander; place them in the bag of breading and shake until well coated. Place the chicken nuggets on the prepared baking sheet, leaving space between them, and bake them 12 to 15 minutes, or until crisp.   *Serves 4*

PER SERVING
EXCHANGES: 1 STARCH, 4 VERY LEAN MEATS, 1½ FATS
NUTRIENTS: 7G FAT/25%, 3.3G SATURATED FAT,
251 CALORIES, 78MG CHOLESTEROL, 481MG SODIUM,
14G CARBOHYDRATE, 31G PROTEIN, 1G DIETARY FIBER

Herbed Turkey Burgers

3 medium scallions
2 garlic cloves
¼ cup packed parsley sprigs
1 pound ground skinless turkey breast
½ cup fine, unseasoned breadcrumbs
2 tablespoons Dijon mustard
2 teaspoons Worcestershire sauce
1 egg white
1 teaspoon dried thyme
¼ teaspoon black pepper
1 tablespoon olive oil

1   In a food processor, mince the scallions, garlic, and parsley.

2   In a medium-size bowl, combine the minced vegetables with the turkey, breadcrumbs, mustard, Worcestershire sauce, egg white, thyme, and pepper and mix to blend well. Divide the mixture into 4 equal portions and form them into patties ½ inch thick.

3   In a large nonstick skillet, warm the oil over medium-high heat until hot but not smoking. Add the turkey patties and cook until well browned on both sides, 3 to 5 minutes for the first side and 2 to 4 minutes for the second side.   *Serves 4*

PER SERVING
EXCHANGES: ¾ STARCH, 4 VERY LEAN MEATS, 1 FAT
NUTRIENTS: 5G FAT/19%, 0.9G SATURATED FAT,
232 CALORIES, 70MG CHOLESTEROL, 398MG SODIUM,
12G CARBOHYDRATE, 31G PROTEIN, 1G DIETARY FIBER

Turkey Scallopini with Vegetables

2 tablespoons flour
1 teaspoon dried basil
½ teaspoon salt
½ teaspoon black pepper
4 turkey cutlets (about 1 pound total),
    pounded thin
1 tablespoon olive oil or other vegetable oil
¼ pound fresh mushrooms, or ½ cup rinsed
    and drained canned mushrooms
1 medium-size yellow squash
1 cup cherry tomatoes, halved
½ cup low-sodium chicken stock

1 In a plastic or paper bag, combine the flour, ½ teaspoon of the basil, and the salt and pepper. Add the turkey cutlets and lightly dredge them in the seasoned flour.

2 In a large nonstick skillet, warm the oil over medium-high heat until hot but not smoking. Add the turkey and cook until light golden on both sides, 3 to 4 minutes per side.

3 Meanwhile, slice the mushrooms ¼ inch thick. Cut the squash into ¼-inch-thick slices.

4 Remove the turkey from the skillet and cover loosely to keep warm. Add the mushrooms, squash, cherry tomatoes, chicken stock, and remaining ½ teaspoon of basil to the skillet. Reduce the heat to medium, cover, and simmer 3 minutes.

5 Return the turkey to the pan. Increase the heat to medium-high, cover, and cook until the turkey is heated through, about 2 minutes.

6 Serve the turkey with the vegetables and some of the pan juices. *Serves 4*

PER SERVING
EXCHANGES: ¼ STARCH, 1 VEGETABLE, 4 VERY LEAN MEATS, 1 FAT
NUTRIENTS: 5G FAT/23%, 0.8G SATURATED FAT, 195 CALORIES, 70MG CHOLESTEROL, 348MG SODIUM, 8G CARBOHYDRATE, 30G PROTEIN, 1G DIETARY FIBER

Spicy Chicken Stew

½ pound acorn squash, peeled and cut into
    ¾-inch dice
1 medium red bell pepper, cut into
    ½-inch-wide strips
2 carrots, cut into ¼-inch diagonal slices
1 cup reduced-sodium chicken stock
1 tablespoon plus 1 teaspoon olive oil
1 medium-size onion, cut into ¼-inch dice
1 pound skinless, boneless chicken breast
3 garlic cloves, minced
One 14-ounce can plum tomatoes,
    with their liquid
1 medium-size zucchini, cut into
    ¼-inch-thick slices
¼ cup golden raisins
¼ teaspoon salt
¼ teaspoon black pepper
⅛ teaspoon ground cinnamon
Dash of hot pepper sauce
½ cup canned chickpeas, rinsed and drained
2 tablespoons sliced toasted almonds
2 teaspoons chopped fresh mint (optional)

1 Place the acorn squash, bell pepper, carrots, and stock in a medium-size saucepan; cover and cook over medium heat 10 minutes, or until the vegetables are crisp-tender; set aside.

2 Heat 2 teaspoons of the oil in a large nonstick skillet over medium-high heat. Add the onion and cook, stirring occasionally, 3 to 5 minutes, or until the onion is golden. Transfer the onion to a plate and set aside.

3 Cut the chicken into ½-inch cubes.

4 Heat the remaining oil in the skillet, then add the chicken and garlic, and cook 5 minutes, or just until the chicken is browned. Transfer the chicken and garlic to the plate with the onion.

5 In the same skillet, combine the tomatoes and their liquid, the zucchini, raisins, salt, black pepper, cinnamon, and hot pepper sauce. Bring the mixture to a boil, breaking up the tomatoes with a spoon, and simmer 5 minutes, or until the vegetables are tender.

6 Add the squash mixture and cook about 4 minutes more to combine the flavors. Return the onion, chicken, and garlic to the skillet, then add the chickpeas and cook 2 minutes, or until the ingredients are heated through.

7 Spoon the stew into 4 bowls and top with the almonds and mint (if using).   *Serves 4*

PER SERVING

EXCHANGES: ½ STARCH, ½ FRUIT, 3½ VEGETABLES, 3½ VERY LEAN MEATS, 1¾ FATS
NUTRIENTS: 9G FAT/25%, 1.3G SATURATED FAT, 329 CALORIES, 66MG CHOLESTEROL, 572MG SODIUM, 31G CARBOHYDRATE, 32G PROTEIN, 7G DIETARY FIBER

◇ ◆ ◇

Skillet Chicken and Vegetables

1⅓ cups brown rice

1 tablespoon plus 1 teaspoon dark sesame oil

3 cups broccoli florets

6 ounces parsnips, cut into 2¼-inch strips

1 medium-size onion, sliced

1 small bell pepper, cut into ¼-inch-wide strips

1½ teaspoons grated fresh ginger

1½ teaspoons minced garlic

1 teaspoon red pepper flakes

10 ounces skinless, boneless chicken breast,
    cut into 2- x ¼-inch strips

4 cups packed spinach leaves

2 cups sliced fresh mushrooms, or ⅔ cup
    rinsed and drained canned mushrooms

¼ cup roasted unsalted cashews

2 tablespoons rice vinegar or
    white wine vinegar

1½ teaspoons reduced-sodium soy sauce

¼ teaspoon salt

1 Bring 3¼ cups of water to a boil in a medium-size saucepan. Stir in the rice, cover, reduce the heat to low, and cook 40 minutes, or until the rice is tender and all of the water is absorbed; remove from the heat and set aside.

2 In a large nonstick skillet or wok, heat 1 tablespoon of the oil over high heat until hot but not smoking. Add the broccoli, parsnips, onion, and bell pepper, and stir-fry 2 minutes, then add the ginger, garlic, and red pepper flakes, and stir-fry another 2 minutes. Using a slotted spoon, transfer the vegetables to a large bowl; set aside.

3 Add the remaining oil to the skillet or wok. Add the chicken and stir-fry 1½ minutes, separating the pieces. Return the cooked vegetables to the skillet and add the spinach, mushrooms, and cashews. Add the vinegar, soy sauce and salt, and stir-fry 2 minutes, or until the mushrooms are just cooked and the spinach is wilted. Divide the rice among 4 plates and spoon the chicken and vegetables on top.   *Serves 4*

PER SERVING

EXCHANGES: 3 STARCHES, 5 VEGETABLES, 2 VERY LEAN MEATS, 2½ FATS
NUTRIENTS: 12G FAT/21%, 2G SATURATED FAT, 507 CALORIES, 41MG CHOLESTEROL, 359MG SODIUM, 73G CARBOHYDRATE, 30G PROTEIN, 11G DIETARY FIBER

Chicken and Vegetable Toss

2 tablespoons wild rice

1 cup brown rice

1 tablespoon cornstarch

¼ teaspoon black pepper

⅛ teaspoon salt

½ pound skinless, boneless chicken breast,
    cut into 2- x ½-inch strips

3 tablespoons butter or margarine

5 shallots, minced

3 garlic cloves, minced

1 tablespoon dry sherry

1 teaspoon dried thyme

2 cups thinly sliced cabbage

2 cups thinly sliced carrots

2 cups thinly sliced zucchini

2 tablespoons chopped fresh dill (optional)

1 Rinse the wild rice in a small strainer under cold running water. In a medium-size saucepan, combine the wild rice, brown rice, and 2 cups of water; bring to a boil over medium-high heat. Cover the pan, reduce the heat to low, and simmer 40 minutes, or until the rice is tender and the water is completely absorbed.

2 Meanwhile, combine the cornstarch, pepper, and salt on a sheet of waxed paper. Gently toss the chicken strips in the cornstarch mixture until coated; set aside.

3 Melt 1½ tablespoons of the butter in a medium-size nonstick skillet over medium-high heat. Add the shallots and half the garlic and sauté 15 seconds. Add the chicken and cook 30 seconds without stirring, then cook, stirring constantly, another 2 to 3 minutes. Add the sherry, half the thyme, and ½ cup of water; cover the pan, reduce the heat to medium-low, and cook 1 minute. Transfer the chicken to a bowl and cover loosely with foil to keep warm. Rinse and dry the skillet.

4 Melt the remaining butter in the skillet over medium-high heat. Add the remaining garlic and thyme, the cabbage, carrots, and zucchini, and cook, stirring constantly, 2 to 3 minutes. Add ¼ cup of water, cover the pan, and cook another minute, or until the cabbage is wilted and the carrots are tender. Return the chicken to the skillet and cook, stirring, 1 minute more.

5 If using the dill, stir it into the rice. Divide the rice among 6 plates and spoon the chicken mixture over it.

Serves 6

PER SERVING

EXCHANGES: 1¾ STARCHES, 2 VEGETABLES,
1 VERY LEAN MEAT, 1½ FATS
NUTRIENTS: 7G FAT/24%, 3.9G SATURATED FAT,
263 CALORIES, 37MG CHOLESTEROL, 152MG SODIUM,
36G CARBOHYDRATE, 13G PROTEIN, 3G DIETARY FIBER

Chicken with Grapes

1¼ cups brown rice

2 shallots, thinly sliced

1 tablespoon olive oil

4 skinless bone-in chicken breast halves
    (about 1½ pounds total weight)

1 cup coarsely chopped celery

½ teaspoon dried thyme

1 bay leaf

Pinch of salt

Pinch of black pepper

¼ cup low-sodium chicken stock

2 cups seedless green grapes

1 teaspoon cornstarch

1 Bring 3 cups of water to a boil in a medium-size saucepan over medium-high heat. Stir in the rice, cover, reduce the heat to low, and simmer 45 minutes, or until the rice is tender and the water is completely absorbed.

2 In a medium-size nonstick skillet over medium heat, sauté the shallots in ½ tablespoon of the olive oil 2 minutes. Add the remaining ½ tablespoon of olive oil to the skillet, then add the chicken breasts and cook about 2 minutes on each side, or until lightly browned.

3 Add the celery, thyme, bay leaf, salt, pepper, and stock. Reduce the heat to low, cover, and simmer the chicken 15 to 20 minutes, or until tender. Add 1½ cups of grapes and simmer another 5 minutes. Remove and discard the bay leaf.

4 In a small bowl, combine the cornstarch with ½ cup cold water and stir well. Stir the cornstarch mixture into the chicken sauce and cook about 2 minutes, or until the sauce is slightly thickened. Divide the rice among 4 plates and place one chicken breast half on each plate. Spoon the sauce and grapes over the chicken and garnish with the remaining grapes.

Serves 4

PER SERVING

EXCHANGES: 2¾ STARCHES, 1 FRUIT, 2 VEGETABLES, 3 VERY LEAN MEATS, 1½ FATS
NUTRIENTS: 7G FAT/13%, 1.4G SATURATED FAT, 478 CALORIES, 76MG CHOLESTEROL, 160MG SODIUM, 66G CARBOHYDRATE, 36G PROTEIN, 4G DIETARY FIBER

Lime Turkey with Fettuccine

1 pound skinless, boneless turkey breast
Grated zest of 1 lime
3 tablespoons lime juice
¼ cup low-sodium chicken stock
1 tablespoon rinsed, drained capers
1 cup golden raisins
¼ teaspoon salt
¼ teaspoon black pepper
½ pound fettuccine
1 tablespoon vegetable oil
2 cups julienne cucumber
2 cups green beans, blanched
1 cup julienne carrots, blanched
1 cup sliced fresh mushrooms
¼ cup chopped fresh parsley (optional)

1 Bring 1 cup of water to a boil in a medium-size skillet over medium heat. Add the turkey, reduce the heat to low, and simmer, uncovered, 15 minutes, or until cooked through. Remove the skillet from the heat and let the turkey cool in the cooking liquid.

2 In a large bowl combine the lime zest, juice, stock, capers, raisins, salt, and pepper. Drain the turkey, place it in the marinade, cover, and refrigerate at least 4 hours, or overnight.

3 Bring a large pot of water to a boil. Cook the fettuccine according to the package directions until al dente; drain, transfer to a large bowl, and toss with the oil. Add the vegetables and toss well.

4 Drain the turkey, reserving the marinade, and cut the turkey on the diagonal into thin slices. Divide the fettuccine mixture among 5 plates and arrange the turkey slices on top. Drizzle with the marinade and sprinkle with parsley (if using).

Serves 5

PER SERVING

EXCHANGES: 2¼ STARCHES, 1½ FRUITS, 1½ VEGETABLES, 2½ VERY LEAN MEATS, 1 FAT
NUTRIENTS: 6G FAT/13%, 1G SATURATED FAT, 421 CALORIES, 99MG CHOLESTEROL, 229MG SODIUM, 63G CARBOHYDRATE, 31G PROTEIN, 5G DIETARY FIBER

BUYING POULTRY

NOT ALL PARTS OF POULTRY ARE CREATED EQUAL WHEN IT COMES TO FAT. THREE AND ONE-HALF OUNCES OF COOKED MEAT FROM CHICKEN WINGS, WITH SKIN, HAVE A WHOPPING 20 GRAMS OF FAT. AN EQUAL PORTION OF SKINLESS BREAST MEAT IS A MUCH WISER CHOICE AT ONLY FOUR GRAMS OF FAT.

Turkey Skillet Dinner

2 cups low-sodium chicken stock

¾ cup white rice

2 tablespoons flour

½ teaspoon salt

¼ teaspoon pepper

½ pound turkey cutlets, cut into
   ¼-inch-wide strips

1 tablespoon olive oil

2 stalks broccoli, cut into bite-size pieces

1 medium-size red onion, thinly sliced

1 cup frozen corn kernels, thawed

3 garlic cloves, minced

3 tablespoons lemon juice

1 teaspoon grated lemon zest

¾ teaspoon dried thyme

1 In a small saucepan, bring 1¾ cups of the stock to a boil. Add the rice, reduce the heat to medium-low, cover, and simmer until tender, 15 to 20 minutes.

2 Meanwhile, in a shallow bowl, combine the flour, salt, and pepper. Lightly dredge the turkey strips in the seasoned flour.

3 In a large nonstick skillet, warm the oil until hot but not smoking. Add the turkey strips and sauté over medium-high heat until cooked through, about 6 minutes. Remove the turkey to a plate.

4 Heat the remaining chicken stock in the skillet over medium-high heat. Add the broccoli, onion, corn, and garlic, and cook 2 minutes.

5 Add the lemon juice, lemon zest, and thyme, and bring to a boil. Reduce the heat to medium-low, cover and simmer until the vegetables are just tender, about 5 minutes.

6 Return the turkey to the skillet, add the cooked rice and toss well to combine.

Serves 4

PER SERVING
EXCHANGES: 2¼ STARCHES, 3 VEGETABLES, 1½ VERY LEAN MEATS, 1 FAT
NUTRIENTS: 6G FAT/16%, 1.1G SATURATED FAT, 328 CALORIES, 35MG CHOLESTEROL, 389MG SODIUM, 50G CARBOHYDRATE, 23G PROTEIN, 4G DIETARY FIBER

Turkey-Mac Chili

One 14-ounce can whole tomatoes,
   with their liquid

1 large green bell pepper, diced

1 medium-size onion, coarsely chopped

½ pound ground skinless turkey breast

2 tablespoons tomato paste

4 garlic cloves, minced

3 tablespoons chili powder

¼ teaspoon black pepper

½ pound elbow macaroni (2 cups)

¼ cup chicken broth

1 tablespoon cornstarch

1 cup canned kidney beans, rinsed and drained

⅓ cup grated cheddar cheese

1 Bring a large pot of water to a boil.

2 Meanwhile, in a medium saucepan, combine the tomatoes and their juice, the bell pepper, onion, turkey, tomato paste, garlic, chili powder, and black pepper. Bring to a boil over medium-high heat, breaking up the tomatoes and turkey with a spoon. Reduce the heat to low, cover, and simmer, stirring occasionally, while you cook the pasta.

3 Add the pasta to the boiling water and cook 10 to 12 minutes, or according to package directions.

4 Meanwhile, in a small bowl, combine the chicken broth and cornstarch. Just before the pasta is done, bring the chili to a boil over medium-high heat. Stir in the broth mixture and the beans and cook, stirring, until the mixture thickens and the beans are heated through, 1 to 2 minutes.

5 Drain the pasta and toss it with the chili. Serve the chili and pasta topped with the cheddar.

Serves 6

PER SERVING
EXCHANGES: 2¼ STARCHES, 2 VEGETABLES, 1¼ VERY LEAN MEATS, ¾ FAT
NUTRIENTS: 4G FAT/12%, 1.5G SATURATED FAT, 295 CALORIES, 30MG CHOLESTEROL, 350MG SODIUM, 45G CARBOHYDRATE, 20G PROTEIN, 6G DIETARY FIBER

Pasta with Turkey-Tomato Sauce

6 garlic cloves
½ pound ground skinless turkey breast
1½ teaspoons dried oregano, crumbled
¾ teaspoon salt
½ teaspoon black pepper
1 tablespoon olive oil
1 medium-size onion, coarsely chopped
One 35-ounce can no-salt-added whole
    tomatoes, with their liquid
2 tablespoons tomato paste
1 bay leaf
½ pound spaghetti

1 Lightly bruise 3 of the garlic cloves; set aside. Mince the remaining 3 garlic cloves.

2 In a small bowl stir together the turkey, minced garlic, ½ teaspoon of the oregano, ½ teaspoon of the salt, and ¼ teaspoon of the pepper.

3 Heat the oil in a medium-size saucepan over medium heat. Add the turkey mixture, onion, and garlic cloves, and cook, stirring to break up the turkey, 3 to 5 minutes, or until the turkey begins to brown.

4 Add the tomatoes with their liquid, the tomato paste, bay leaf, and remaining oregano, salt, and pepper. Bring the mixture to a boil, breaking up the tomatoes with a spoon. Reduce the heat to medium-low and simmer 20 minutes, stirring occasionally.

5 About 15 minutes before the sauce is done, remove and discard garlic cloves and bay leaf. Bring a large pot of water to a boil. Cook the spaghetti 10 to 12 minutes, or according to the package directions.

6 Drain the spaghetti and divide it among 4 plates. Spoon some sauce over each serving.   *Serves 4*

PER SERVING

EXCHANGES: 2¾ STARCHES, 4 VEGETABLES,
1 VERY LEAN MEAT, 1 FAT
NUTRIENTS: 5G FAT/12%, 0.8G SATURATED FAT,
386 CALORIES, 35MG CHOLESTEROL, 543MG SODIUM,
60G CARBOHYDRATE, 25G PROTEIN, 5G DIETARY FIBER

Ziti with Chicken and Peppers

3 cups low-sodium chicken stock
1 cup water
2 garlic cloves, minced
3 drops hot pepper sauce
¼ to ½ teaspoon red pepper flakes, to taste
¼ teaspoon black pepper
2 large sweet potatoes (1 pound total)
½ pound ziti or wagon-wheel pasta
1 large green bell pepper
½ pound skinless, boneless chicken breast
3 tablespoons grated Parmesan cheese

1 In a large skillet, combine the chicken stock, water, garlic, hot pepper sauce, red pepper flakes, and black pepper, and bring to a boil over medium-high heat.

2 Meanwhile, peel the sweet potatoes and cut into ¼-inch dice.

3 When the broth has come to a boil, add the sweet potatoes and pasta. Stir and return the liquid to a boil. Reduce the heat to medium-low, cover, and simmer about 7 minutes, or until the pasta is done.

4 Meanwhile, cut the bell pepper into thin strips. Cut the chicken across the grain into ¼-inch-wide strips.

5 Return the mixture in the skillet to a boil over medium-high heat. Stir in the bell pepper and chicken. Let the mixture return to a boil, then reduce heat to medium-low, cover, and simmer, stirring occasionally, until the chicken is cooked through, 5 to 7 minutes.

6 Stir in the Parmesan and serve.   *Serves 6*

PER SERVING

EXCHANGES: 2¾ STARCHES, ¼ VEGETABLE,
1 VERY LEAN MEAT, ½ FAT
NUTRIENTS: 3G FAT/10%, 1G SATURATED FAT,
269 CALORIES, 24MG CHOLESTEROL, 140MG SODIUM,
44G CARBOHYDRATE, 17G PROTEIN, 3G DIETARY FIBER

Chicken Pot Pie

½ cup unbleached all-purpose flour
Pinch of salt
2 tablespoons chopped fresh dill, or
   2 teaspoons dried dill
2 tablespoons margarine, well chilled
1 tablespoon ice water
1 cup low-sodium chicken stock
3 cups unpeeled, diced new potatoes
1 cup chopped onions
3 cups broccoli florets
1 cup canned or frozen corn kernels
1 tablespoon cornstarch
½ pound skinless cooked chicken breast, cut
   into large chunks

1   Place all but 1 tablespoon of the flour in a small bowl. Add the salt and 1 tablespoon of the fresh dill (or 1 teaspoon of dried dill), and stir well to combine.

2   Using a pastry blender or two knives, cut the margarine into the dry ingredients until the mixture resembles coarse cornmeal. Add the ice water and stir until the dough forms a ball. Cover the bowl with a kitchen towel and set aside.

3   Bring the stock to a boil in a medium-size saucepan over medium heat. Add the potatoes and onions and return the mixture to a boil. Reduce the heat to medium-low, cover the pan, and simmer the vegetables 10 to 15 minutes, or until the potatoes are tender when pierced with a knife.

4   Preheat the oven to 400°.

5   Uncover the pan of potatoes, add the broccoli and corn, and return the mixture to a boil.

6   In a small bowl stir together the cornstarch and ¼ cup of cold water until smooth. Add the chicken to the saucepan, then stir in the cornstarch mixture and simmer 1 to 2 minutes, or until the sauce thickens. Stir in the remaining dill. Turn the chicken mixture into a shallow 10-inch baking dish and set aside.

7   Remove the dough from the bowl and place it on a lightly floured work surface. With your hands, flatten the ball of dough into a disk; then, using a lightly floured rolling pin, roll it out ¼ inch thick. Place the dough on top of the chicken mixture and bake 15 to 20 minutes, or until the crust is golden.   *Serves 4*

PER SERVING

EXCHANGES: 3 STARCHES, 1¾ VEGETABLES,
2 VERY LEAN MEATS, 2 FATS
NUTRIENTS: 9G FAT/21%, 1.8G SATURATED FAT,
394 CALORIES, 48MG CHOLESTEROL, 348MG SODIUM,
54G CARBOHYDRATE, 27G PROTEIN, 7G DIETARY FIBER

Sautéed Chicken with Peppers

1 lemon
1 pound skinless, boneless chicken breast
   halves
2 tablespoons flour
¼ teaspoon salt
⅛ teaspoon black pepper
1 tablespoon plus 1 teaspoon olive oil
1 garlic clove, crushed
3 bell peppers (preferably red, green, and
   yellow), cut into ¼-inch-wide strips
⅓ cup dry white wine
½ cup low-sodium chicken stock
2 teaspoons cornstarch
1 tablespoon finely chopped parsley (optional)

1   Halve the lemon and slice one half; squeeze 1 tablespoon of juice from the other half.

2   Cut the chicken breasts in half crosswise and pound gently to flatten them. Sprinkle the chicken with flour, salt, and pepper, and pat in the coating.

3   Heat the oil and garlic in a large nonstick skillet over medium-high heat until the oil is hot but not smoking. Discard the garlic. Add a single layer of chicken pieces to the skillet, increase the heat to high, and sauté about 1 minute on each side, or until golden brown. Transfer the cooked chicken to a platter and cover loosely to keep warm. Sauté the remaining chicken and transfer it to the platter.

4   Add the peppers, wine, and lemon juice to the skillet, and cook, covered, over medium-low heat 5 minutes, or until the peppers are slightly softened. Uncover and cook over high heat 5 minutes to reduce the sauce to about 2 tablespoons.

5 Stir together the stock and cornstarch, then stir this mixture into the sauce. Bring to a boil and cook 1 minute. Stir in the parsley (if using). Pour the sauce and peppers over the chicken and garnish with the reserved lemon slices.   *Serves 4*

PER SERVING

EXCHANGES: ½ STARCH, 1 VEGETABLE, 3½ VERY LEAN MEATS, 1¼ FATS
NUTRIENTS: 6G FAT/25%, 1.1G SATURATED FAT, 219 CALORIES, 66MG CHOLESTEROL, 226MG SODIUM, 10G CARBOHYDRATE, 28G PROTEIN, 1G DIETARY FIBER

◇ ◇ ◇

Baked Chicken and Vegetables

2 skinless, boneless chicken breast halves
½ cup plain lowfat yogurt
1 tablespoon lemon juice
1 teaspoon curry powder
½ teaspoon ground cumin
⅛ teaspoon ground red pepper
½ teaspoon salt
½ teaspoon black pepper
2 large baking potatoes (1 pound total)
1 large sweet potato
½ pound carrots
½ pound onions
5 garlic cloves
1½ tablespoons olive oil

1 Cut each chicken breast into two pieces.

2 In a glass bowl stir together the yogurt, lemon juice, curry powder, cumin, ground red pepper, ¼ teaspoon of the salt, and ¼ teaspoon of the black pepper. Add the chicken, turning it to coat evenly with the marinade. Cover the bowl with plastic wrap and let marinate in the refrigerator at least 1 hour and up to 24 hours.

3 Meanwhile, wash and peel the baking potatoes

and sweet potato. Wash and trim the carrots; peel the onions and garlic cloves. Cut the potatoes, carrots, and onions into 1-inch pieces; mince the garlic cloves; set aside.

4 Preheat the oven to 400°.

5 Combine the vegetables in a large baking dish, sprinkle them with the oil and the remaining salt and pepper, and toss to coat the vegetables with oil. Bake 30 minutes, or until the potatoes are softened.

6 Add the chicken and marinade to the baking dish and stir to combine. Cover the dish with foil, reduce the oven temperature to 350°, and bake another 30 minutes, or until the chicken is tender. Transfer the chicken and vegetables to a serving dish.   *Serves 4*

PER SERVING

EXCHANGES: 2 STARCHES, 2½ VEGETABLES, 1½ VERY LEAN MEATS, 1½ FATS
NUTRIENTS: 7G FAT/20%, 1.2G SATURATED FAT, 315 CALORIES, 36MG CHOLESTEROL, 368MG SODIUM, 45G CARBOHYDRATE, 19G PROTEIN, 6G DIETARY FIBER

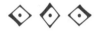

◇ ◇ ◇

HANDLING POULTRY

REFRIGERATE RAW POULTRY IN ITS ORIGINAL WRAPPING FOR UP TO TWO DAYS OR FREEZE, OVERWRAPPED WITH PLASTIC WRAP OR FOIL, FOR UP TO TWO MONTHS. THAW FROZEN POULTRY OVERNIGHT IN THE REFRIGERATOR, NEVER AT ROOM TEMPERATURE. TO PREVENT ANY BACTERIA PRESENT IN RAW POULTRY FROM SPREADING TO OTHER FOODS, DO NOT LET THE POULTRY COME IN CONTACT WITH FOODS, AND WASH WORK SURFACES, UTENSILS, AND HANDS WITH HOT, SOAPY WATER AFTER HANDLING POULTRY.

Curried Turkey Salad

½ cup fat-free mayonnaise
½ cup plain lowfat yogurt
¼ cup buttermilk
1 tablespoon apricot fruit spread
1½ teaspoons curry powder
⅛ teaspoon ground ginger
3 cups skinless cooked turkey breast, cut into 1-inch cubes
One 13¼-ounce can juice-packed pineapple chunks, drained
1 cup thinly sliced celery
¼ cup thinly sliced scallions
½ cup frozen green peas, thawed
1 Granny Smith or other tart green apple, peeled, cored, and diced
Small head leaf lettuce
¾ ounce fresh or frozen snow peas, blanched

1 Combine the mayonnaise, yogurt, buttermilk, fruit spread, curry powder, and ginger in a small bowl; set aside.

2 In a large bowl combine the turkey, pineapple, celery, scallions, peas, and apple. Add the dressing and toss to combine. Refrigerate the salad at least 2 hours, or until well chilled.

3 To serve, line a platter with lettuce and spoon the turkey salad on top. Top with snow peas. *Serves 4*

PER SERVING

EXCHANGES: ¼ LOWFAT MILK, 1 OTHER CARBOHYDRATE, 1 VEGETABLE, 4 VERY LEAN MEATS, 1¼ FRUITS
NUTRIENTS: 2G FAT/5%, 0.7G SATURATED FAT, 334 CALORIES, 91MG CHOLESTEROL, 387MG SODIUM, 43G CARBOHYDRATE, 36G PROTEIN, 3G DIETARY FIBER

Lemon Chicken Salad

1 pound skinless, boneless chicken breast
¼ cup plain nonfat yogurt
2 tablespoons mayonnaise
¼ cup lemon juice
2 teaspoons grated lemon zest (optional)
½ teaspoon salt
¼ teaspoon black pepper
¼ teaspoon cayenne pepper
3 quarter-size slices (¼ inch thick) fresh ginger, unpeeled
¼ cup parsley sprigs (optional)
1 large carrot
4 scallions
1 large green bell pepper
1 pint cherry tomatoes

1 Place the chicken in a vegetable steamer over boiling water and steam until cooked through, about 12 minutes. Remove the chicken to a plate and cover loosely to keep warm.

2 Meanwhile, in a salad bowl, combine the yogurt, mayonnaise, lemon juice, lemon zest (if using), salt, black pepper, and cayenne pepper.

3 In a food processor, mince the ginger and parsley (if using). Add the mixture to the salad bowl.

4 In the same processor work bowl, finely chop the carrot and scallions and add them to the salad bowl.

5 Cut the bell pepper into thin strips. Halve the cherry tomatoes. Add the bell pepper and tomatoes to the salad bowl.

6 When the chicken is cool enough to handle, shred it and add it to the bowl of vegetables. Toss the ingredients to coat with the dressing. *Serves 4*

PER SERVING

EXCHANGES: 2 VEGETABLES, 3½ VERY LEAN MEATS, 1½ FATS
NUTRIENTS: 7G FAT/29%, 1.2G SATURATED FAT, 221 CALORIES, 70MG CHOLESTEROL, 418MG SODIUM, 10G CARBOHYDRATE, 28G PROTEIN, 2G DIETARY FIBER

Vegetable, Chicken, and Cheese Melt

1 tablespoon olive oil
1 cup chopped onion
2 garlic cloves, minced
3 red bell peppers, seeded and coarsely diced
2 medium-size zucchini, sliced ¼ inch thick
Black pepper
¼ pound skinless, boneless chicken breast,
    cut into ½-inch chunks
Four 2-ounce whole-wheat pita breads
½ cup shredded part-skim mozzarella
3 cups shredded fresh spinach or watercress

1 Heat 2½ teaspoons of the oil in a medium-size nonstick skillet over medium heat. Add the onion and garlic, and cook, stirring, 4 minutes. Increase the heat to medium-high, add the bell peppers and zucchini, and cook, stirring, 5 minutes. Add ½ cup of water and cook 3 minutes more. Add black pepper to taste. Using a slotted spoon, transfer the vegetables to a bowl to cool. Add the chicken to the skillet and cook, stirring, over medium heat 5 minutes, or until cooked through. Transfer the chicken to a small bowl. Wipe the skillet with paper towels; set aside.

2 Split the pita breads and sprinkle the bottom halves with mozzarella. Divide the vegetable mixture, chicken, and spinach among the sandwiches and cover with the top halves of the pita breads.

3 Brush the skillet with the remaining oil and heat over medium-high heat. Place one sandwich at a time in the skillet and heat it 3 minutes, or until the cheese melts, then carefully turn and heat it 2 minutes longer. *Serves 4*

PER SERVING

EXCHANGES: 2 STARCHES, 2 VEGETABLES, 1 VERY LEAN MEAT, 1½ FATS
NUTRIENTS: 8G FAT/24%, 2.2G SATURATED FAT, 295 CALORIES, 25MG CHOLESTEROL, 402MG SODIUM, 42G CARBOHYDRATE, 18G PROTEIN, 7G DIETARY FIBER

Chicken Club with Carrot Salad

1½ tablespoons lowfat mayonnaise
1½ tablespoons plain lowfat yogurt
1½ cups shredded carrots
⅓ cup raisins
1 teaspoon lemon juice
½ teaspoon grated lemon zest
1 tablespoon spicy brown mustard
1 ounce Canadian bacon
4 leaves romaine lettuce
1 medium-size tomato, sliced
½ medium-size onion, sliced
2 ounces thinly sliced cooked chicken breast
6 slices whole-wheat bread

1 Mix the mayonnaise and yogurt in a cup.

2 In a small bowl, stir together the carrots, raisins, lemon juice, lemon zest, and half the mayonnaise mixture. Stir the mustard into the remaining mayonnaise mixture. Cover both bowls and refrigerate.

3 Cook the bacon in a small nonstick skillet over medium heat 1 minute on each side, or until heated through; set aside.

4 Divide the romaine, tomato, and onion into 4 portions and the chicken and bacon into 2 portions; set aside. Toast the bread and spread one side of each slice with the mayonnaise mixture.

5 To assemble each sandwich, top a slice of toast with a portion of romaine, tomato, onion, and chicken; place another slice of toast on top. Add another portion of romaine, tomato, and onion, and top with bacon and the last slice of toast. Insert 2 long toothpicks or small skewers into each sandwich. Using a serrated knife, cut the sandwiches diagonally in half. Serve with the salad. *Serves 2*

PER SERVING

EXCHANGES: 3 STARCHES, 1¼ FRUITS, 3 VEGETABLES, 1 VERY LEAN MEAT, 1½ FATS
NUTRIENTS: 8G FAT/16%, 1.6G SATURATED FAT, 457 CALORIES, 32MG CHOLESTEROL, 900MG SODIUM, 79G CARBOHYDRATE, 25G PROTEIN, 12G DIETARY FIBER

Chicken, Potato, and Carrot Stew

2 tablespoons flour
½ teaspoon salt
¼ teaspoon black pepper
8 chicken drumsticks (about 2 pounds total), skinned
1 tablespoon vegetable oil
10 garlic cloves, peeled
4 carrots, thinly sliced
2 bunches scallions, cut into 2-inch lengths
1½ pounds red potatoes, thinly sliced
1½ teaspoons dried rosemary
1 cup dry white wine
2 cups reduced-sodium chicken stock
1½ cups frozen peas

1 On a plate, combine the flour, ¼ teaspoon of the salt, and the pepper. Dredge the chicken in the flour mixture, shaking off the excess. In a large, heavy non-stick saucepan, heat the oil over medium heat until hot but not smoking. Add the chicken and cook for 5 minutes, or until golden brown on all sides. Transfer the chicken to a plate.

2 Add the garlic, carrots, scallions, potatoes, rosemary, and the remaining ¼ teaspoon salt to the pan and cook, stirring frequently, for 5 minutes, or until the vegetables begin to brown. Add the wine and cook for 3 minutes. Return the chicken to the pan and add the stock. Bring to a boil over medium-high heat, reduce to a simmer, and cover. Cook, turning the chicken occasionally, for 15 minutes, or until the meat is cooked through and the vegetables are tender.

3 Stir in the peas and cook, uncovered, for 3 minutes longer, or until the peas are heated through. Spoon the stew into 4 bowls and serve.   *Serves 4*

PER SERVING
EXCHANGES: 2¾ STARCHES, 1 OTHER CARBOHYDRATE, 2 VEGETABLES, 3¼ VERY LEAN MEATS, 1 FAT
NUTRIENTS: 8G FAT/15%, 1.6G SATURATED FAT, 481 CALORIES, 94MG CHOLESTEROL, 816MG SODIUM, 57G CARBOHYDRATE, 36G PROTEIN, 9G DIETARY FIBER

Turkey Sandwich with 3-Fruit Relish

1 small apple, washed and cored
1 small seedless orange, washed
½ cup cranberries
1 tablespoon frozen unsweetened apple juice concentrate, thawed
1 cup sliced fresh mushrooms, or ⅓ cup rinsed and drained canned mushrooms
8 slices whole-wheat bread
1 tablespoon soft margarine
¼ pound skinless cooked turkey breast, thinly sliced
1 cup grated carrots
2 tomatoes, sliced
2 cups romaine lettuce, torn into bite-size pieces

1 For the relish, cut the apple and orange into large chunks and place them in a food processor or blender. Add the cranberries and apple juice, and process, pulsing the machine on and off, about 20 seconds, or until the fruit is coarsely chopped and well mixed; set aside.

2 In a small nonstick skillet, cook the mushrooms with 1 tablespoon of water over medium heat, stirring often, 3 to 5 minutes, or until softened.

3 Spread one side of each slice of bread with margarine. Divide the turkey among 4 slices of bread and top it with mushrooms, carrots, tomatoes, and romaine. Spread the remaining slices of bread with relish and place them on top of the sandwiches. (If making the sandwiches ahead of time, do not add the relish until just before serving, or it will soak through the bread.) Cut the sandwiches in half and serve.

Serves 4

PER SERVING
EXCHANGES: 2 STARCHES, ¾ FRUIT, ¾ VEGETABLE, 1 VERY LEAN MEAT, 1¼ FATS
NUTRIENTS: 6G FAT/19%, 1.1G SATURATED FAT, 278 CALORIES, 24MG CHOLESTEROL, 372MG SODIUM, 45G CARBOHYDRATE, 16G PROTEIN, 7G DIETARY FIBER

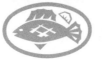

Sole in Packets

1 tablespoon plus 1 teaspoon butter

⅓ cup sliced scallions

2 teaspoons lemon juice

1 garlic clove, minced

¼ teaspoon salt

⅛ teaspoon paprika

⅛ teaspoon black pepper

Dash of hot pepper sauce

½ pound fillet of sole, cut into 4 equal pieces

6 small unpeeled red potatoes, boiled and
    sliced ¼ inch thick

6 ounces snow peas, trimmed and blanched

1 Preheat the oven to 350°.

2 Melt the butter in a small saucepan over low heat. Stir in the scallions, lemon juice, garlic, salt, paprika, pepper, and hot pepper sauce. Cook 2 to 3 minutes, or until fragrant; set aside.

3 Cut four 12-inch squares of heavy-duty aluminum foil. Place a portion of sole on one side of each sheet of foil and divide the potatoes and snow peas among the four portions. Spoon the butter mixture over the fish and vegetables. Fold the foil over the food and firmly crimp the edges to seal the packets. Place the packets on a baking sheet and bake 12 minutes, or until the fish flakes when tested with a fork (open one packet to test for doneness).

4 Place each packet on a plate and open the packets just before serving.   *Serves 4*

PER SERVING

EXCHANGES: 1¾ STARCHES, 1½ VEGETABLES,
1 VERY LEAN MEAT, 1 FAT
NUTRIENTS: 5G FAT/18%, 2.6G SATURATED FAT,
246 CALORIES, 38MG CHOLESTEROL, 239MG SODIUM,
35G CARBOHYDRATE, 15G PROTEIN, 4G DIETARY FIBER

Flounder with Spinach and Garlic

1 pound flounder or sole fillets

½ teaspoon dried tarragon, crumbled

½ teaspoon black pepper

¼ teaspoon salt

2 teaspoons olive oil

3 garlic cloves, peeled and thinly sliced

1 pound spinach, torn into bite-size pieces

½ cup chicken stock

1½ teaspoons fresh lemon juice

1 lemon, cut into 8 wedges

1 Cut the fish fillets in half lengthwise, then cut crosswise into 1½-inch-wide pieces. Sprinkle the fish with the tarragon, ¼ teaspoon of the pepper, and ⅛ teaspoon of the salt.

2 Heat the oil a large nonstick skillet over medium-high heat until hot but not smoking. Add the garlic and sauté just until light golden, about 1 minute. Add the spinach by handfuls, adding more as it wilts. When all the spinach is wilted, add the stock and the remaining ¼ teaspoon pepper and ⅛ teaspoon salt; bring to a boil over high heat. Reduce the heat to low, cover, and simmer, stirring occasionally, until the spinach is tender, 2 to 3 minutes.

3 Arrange the pieces of fish in a single layer over the spinach. Cover and cook over medium heat until the fish barely flakes when tested with a fork, about 5 minutes. Remove from the heat.

4 Drizzle the fish and spinach with the lemon juice. Spoon into 4 shallow plates and serve with the lemon wedges.   *Serves 4*

PER SERVING

EXCHANGES: ¼ STARCH, 1 VEGETABLE,
3 VERY LEAN MEATS, ¾ FAT
NUTRIENTS: 4G FAT/22%, 0.7G SATURATED FAT,
162 CALORIES, 54MG CHOLESTEROL, 443MG SODIUM,
8G CARBOHYDRATE, 25G PROTEIN, 3G DIETARY FIBER

Baked Fish with Oven Fries

1¼ pounds baking potatoes
1 tablespoon plus 1 teaspoon vegetable oil
½ teaspoon dried basil
½ teaspoon dried oregano
½ teaspoon black pepper
¼ teaspoon salt
½ teaspoon paprika
1 pound skinned haddock fillets, cut into
    4 equal pieces
1½ teaspoons fresh lemon juice

1 Preheat the oven to 450°. Spray a heavy baking sheet and a 13- x 9-inch baking dish with nonstick cooking spray.

2 Cut the unpeeled potatoes lengthwise into thin (¼-inch) sticks. Pile the potatoes in the center of the prepared baking sheet and toss with the oil.

3 In a small bowl, mix the basil, oregano, pepper, and salt. Sprinkle half of this mixture on the potatoes and toss until well coated. Spread the potatoes into a single layer on the baking sheet.

4 Mix the paprika into the remaining basil mixture. Place the haddock in the baking dish. Drizzle with the lemon juice and sprinkle with the basil mixture.

5 Bake the potatoes until lightly browned on the underside, about 18 minutes. Use a large spatula to turn the potatoes, then bake another 10 minutes.

6 Place the fish in the oven. Bake until the potatoes are browned and crisp and the fish just flakes when tested with a fork, about 10 minutes.

7 Serve the oven fries with the fish.

Serves 4

PER SERVING
EXCHANGES: 1¾ STARCHES, 3 VERY LEAN MEATS, 1 FAT
NUTRIENTS: 6G FAT/21%, 0.7G SATURATED FAT,
260 CALORIES, 65MG CHOLESTEROL, 223MG SODIUM,
26G CARBOHYDRATE, 24G PROTEIN, 2G DIETARY FIBER

Fish Steaks with Pineapple Sauce

1 small red onion
One 8-ounce can juice-packed crushed
    pineapple
3 garlic cloves, minced
3 tablespoons ketchup
2 tablespoons chopped scallion greens
2 teaspoons cornstarch
½ teaspoon salt
¼ teaspoon hot pepper flakes
Pinch of ground red pepper
Four 1-inch-thick tuna steaks (1 pound total)

1 Coarsely chop the onion.

2 In a medium-size saucepan, combine the chopped onion, the pineapple and its juice, the garlic, ketchup, scallion greens, cornstarch, salt, hot pepper flakes, and ground red pepper. Bring to a boil over medium heat, stirring frequently. Cook, uncovered, 10 minutes, stirring occasionally.

3 Reduce the heat to low and simmer, uncovered, until thickened, about 10 minutes.

4 Meanwhile, preheat the broiler. Line a broiler pan with foil and lightly spray with nonstick cooking spray.

5 Place the steaks on the broiler pan. Top each steak with one-fourth of the pineapple sauce and broil 4 inches from the heat 12 minutes, or until the fish just flakes when tested with the tip of a knife.

Serves 4

PER SERVING
EXCHANGES: ½ FRUIT, 1½ VEGETABLES,
3 VERY LEAN MEATS, 1¼ FATS
NUTRIENTS: 6G FAT/23%, 1.4G SATURATED FAT,
233 CALORIES, 43MG CHOLESTEROL, 457MG SODIUM,
17G CARBOHYDRATE, 28G PROTEIN, 1G DIETARY FIBER

Stuffed Trout

½ cup low-sodium chicken stock

2 tablespoons margarine

2 cups diced red bell pepper

1½ cups sliced fresh mushrooms, or ½ cup
    rinsed and drained canned mushrooms

1 cup fresh or frozen corn kernels

1 cup sliced yellow squash

1 cup chopped scallions

2 garlic cloves, chopped

5 cups whole-wheat bread cubes

One 1½-pound brook trout, cleaned

1 lemon

1 Preheat the oven to 400°.

2 For the stuffing, bring the stock to a boil in a large skillet over medium-high heat. Add the margarine, bell pepper, mushrooms, corn, squash, scallions, and garlic, and cook, stirring constantly, until the mixture returns to a boil. Remove the skillet from the heat and stir in the bread cubes until thoroughly combined; set aside.

3 Rinse the trout and pat it dry with paper towels. Transfer three-fourths of the stuffing to a large, shallow baking pan and pat it into an even layer. Place the trout on top and fill the cavity of the fish with the remaining stuffing. Cover the pan with foil and bake 20 to 25 minutes, or until the fish flakes when tested with a fork.

4 Halve the lemon and squeeze the juice of one half over the trout; slice the other half and use it to garnish the fish.

Serves 4

PER SERVING

EXCHANGES: 1¾ STARCHES, ¼ FRUIT, 1½ VEGETABLES, 3 VERY LEAN MEATS, 2½ FATS
NUTRIENTS: 12G FAT/30%, 2.2G SATURATED FAT, 361 CALORIES, 60MG CHOLESTEROL, 354MG SODIUM, 39G CARBOHYDRATE, 30G PROTEIN, 6G DIETARY FIBER

Halibut with Cucumber-Chive Sauce

1 tablespoon butter or margarine

¼ cup snipped fresh chives or scallions

½ teaspoon salt

½ teaspoon black pepper

4 small halibut fillets (1 pound total)

½ cup nonfat sour cream

½ cup plain lowfat yogurt

3 tablespoons lemon juice

2 teaspoons grated lemon zest (optional)

½ teaspoon dry mustard

¼ cup peeled, finely chopped cucumber

¼ cup minced red bell pepper

1 Preheat the broiler. Line a broiler pan with foil and spray the foil with nonstick cooking spray.

2 Melt the butter in a small saucepan.

3 In a small bowl, combine the melted butter with 1 tablespoon of the chives, ¼ teaspoon of the salt, and ¼ teaspoon of the black pepper.

4 Place the fish on the broiler pan. Spread the chive mixture over the fish and broil 4 inches from the heat until the fish is opaque and just flakes when tested with the tip of a knife, about 7 minutes.

5 Meanwhile, in a medium-size bowl, combine the sour cream, yogurt, lemon juice, lemon zest (if using), mustard, the remaining 3 tablespoons chives, ¼ teaspoon salt, and ¼ teaspoon black pepper. Stir in the cucumber and bell pepper.

6 Serve the fish with the cucumber-chive sauce.

Serves 4

PER SERVING

EXCHANGES: 1 VEGETABLE, 1¼ FATS, 3 VERY LEAN MEATS
NUTRIENTS: 6G FAT/27%, 2.4G SATURATED FAT, 198 CALORIES, 46MG CHOLESTEROL, 407MG SODIUM, 6G CARBOHYDRATE, 27G PROTEIN, 0G DIETARY FIBER

Crispy Sweet-and-Sour Cod

½ cup plain lowfat yogurt

1 tablespoon peach fruit spread

2 teaspoons Dijon mustard

1 teaspoon cider vinegar

1 tablespoon chopped parsley (optional)

1 egg white

2 tablespoons lowfat (1%) milk

¾ cup fine, unseasoned breadcrumbs

¼ cup grated Parmesan cheese

½ teaspoon salt

¼ teaspoon black pepper

1 pound cod fillets (about ½ inch thick)

1 In a medium-size bowl, combine the yogurt, peach spread, mustard, vinegar, and parsley (if using), and stir to blend.

2 Preheat the oven to 400°.

3 Line a baking sheet with foil and lightly spray with nonstick cooking spray.

4 In a shallow bowl, beat the egg white and milk together. In another shallow bowl, combine the breadcrumbs, Parmesan, salt, and pepper.

5 Dip the fish first into the egg mixture and then into the breadcrumbs, coating well on both sides.

6 Place the fish on the prepared baking sheet in a single layer. Bake, uncovered, 10 to 12 minutes, or until the fish is opaque and flakes easily when tested with the tip of a knife.

7 Serve the fish with the sweet-and-sour sauce on the side.

Serves 4

PER SERVING

EXCHANGES: 1 STARCH, ¼ LOWFAT MILK, ½ FAT, 3 VERY LEAN MEATS
NUTRIENTS: 4G FAT/15%, 1.7G SATURATED FAT, 236 CALORIES, 55MG CHOLESTEROL, 700MG SODIUM, 20G CARBOHYDRATE, 27G PROTEIN, 1G DIETARY FIBER

Flounder Rolls with Cheese and Spinach

3 garlic cloves

3 medium scallions, cut into 2-inch pieces

5 ounces frozen chopped spinach, thawed

½ cup part-skim ricotta cheese

¼ cup reduced-fat grated Swiss cheese

1 tablespoon grated Parmesan cheese

1 egg white

2 teaspoons grated lemon zest (optional)

3 tablespoons flour

1 teaspoon oregano

¼ teaspoon black pepper

4 flounder or sole fillets (1 pound total)

¼ cup lemon juice

2 teaspoons margarine

1 Preheat the oven to 350°. Spray an 11- x 7-inch baking dish with nonstick cooking spray.

2 In a food processor, mince the garlic. Add the scallions and chop finely.

3 Place the spinach between several sheets of paper towels and squeeze it as dry as possible.

4 In a medium-size bowl, combine the garlic-scallion mixture, the spinach, ricotta, Swiss cheese, Parmesan, egg white, lemon zest (if using), flour, oregano, and pepper.

5 Place the fillets on a work surface. Dividing evenly, spread each fillet with the filling. Loosely roll up the fillets and place them seam side down in the prepared baking dish.

6 Pour the lemon juice over the fish and dot each roll with ½ teaspoon of the margarine. Bake the fish 20 minutes, or until the fish just flakes when tested with a fork. About halfway through the baking, spoon some of the pan juices over the fish.

Serves 4

PER SERVING

EXCHANGES: ¼ STARCH, 1¼ VEGETABLE, 4 VERY LEAN MEATS, 1½ FATS
NUTRIENTS: 8G FAT/30%, 3G SATURATED FAT, 238 CALORIES, 69MG CHOLESTEROL, 234MG SODIUM, 10G CARBOHYDRATE, 31G PROTEIN, 1G DIETARY FIBER

Linguine with Tuna Sauce

1 tablespoon olive oil
¼ cup chopped onion
1 garlic clove, crushed
One 12-ounce can crushed tomatoes
One 12½-ounce can water-packed tuna, drained
¼ cup black olives, slivered
2 tablespoons red wine
1 small bay leaf
¼ teaspoon dried oregano, crumbled
¼ teaspoon red pepper flakes
12 ounces linguine or fettuccine
2 tablespoons chopped fresh parsley (optional)

1 Heat the oil in a large saucepan. Add the onion and cook until translucent. Add the garlic and brown slightly. Add all the remaining ingredients except the linguine and parsley (if using) and bring to a boil. Reduce the heat and simmer 20 minutes. Remove and discard the bay leaf.

2 Bring a large saucepan of water to a boil. Cook the linguine 8 to 10 minutes, or according to package directions.

3 Drain the linguine in a colander, then transfer it to 4 plates. Top with the sauce and sprinkle with the chopped parsley (if using).

Serves 4

PER SERVING

EXCHANGES: 4 STARCHES, 2 VEGETABLES, 2¾ VERY LEAN MEATS, 1¼ FATS
NUTRIENTS: 6G FAT/11%, 0.9G SATURATED FAT, 487 CALORIES, 33MG CHOLESTEROL, 500MG SODIUM, 69G CARBOHYDRATE, 35G PROTEIN, 3G DIETARY FIBER

Tex-Mex Steamed Snapper

2 red snapper fillets (about 1¼ pounds total)
2 cups spinach leaves
1 large red bell pepper, cut into thin rings
1 medium-size red onion, cut into thin rings
2 limes
1 tablespoon vegetable oil
1 teaspoon chili powder
¾ teaspoon cumin
¼ teaspoon red pepper flakes
¼ teaspoon salt
¼ teaspoon black pepper
Eight 5½-inch corn tortillas

1 Cut the fillets in half to make 4 equal portions.

2 Line a flat vegetable steamer with the spinach, bell pepper, and onion. Steam the vegetables over boiling water about 1 minute.

3 Meanwhile, grate the zest from one of the limes. Cut both limes into quarters.

4 In a bowl combine the oil, lime zest, chili powder, cumin, red pepper flakes, salt, and black pepper.

5 Remove the steamer from the heat. Place the fish skin side down on top of the steamed vegetables. Brush the fish with the seasoned oil. Re-cover and steam until the fish just flakes when tested with a fork, about 4 minutes.

6 Meanwhile, wrap the tortillas in foil and warm them in the oven or a toaster oven. Or wrap them in a damp paper towel and warm in a microwave.

7 Dividing evenly, serve the fish with the steamed vegetables. Using one-quarter lime per portion, squeeze the lime juice over the fish. Serve with 1 lime wedge and 2 tortillas per person.

Serves 4

PER SERVING

EXCHANGES: 1¾ STARCHES, ¼ FRUIT, ½ VEGETABLE, 4 VERY LEAN MEATS, 1½ FATS
NUTRIENTS: 7G FAT/19%, 1G SATURATED FAT, 325 CALORIES, 52MG CHOLESTEROL, 341MG SODIUM, 33G CARBOHYDRATE, 34G PROTEIN, 5G DIETARY FIBER

Mediterranean-Style Tuna Salad

¾ pound small red potatoes
5 ounces green beans, cut into 1½-inch pieces
   (1 cup)
¼ cup red wine vinegar
1 tablespoon olive oil
1 tablespoon Dijon mustard
1 tablespoon chopped fresh chives
Pinch of salt
Pinch of black pepper
2 medium-size tomatoes
8 ounces romaine lettuce, torn into pieces
Two 6⅛-ounce cans water-packed
   white tuna, drained

1 Bring a medium-size saucepan of water to a boil. Scrub the potatoes and place them in the boiling water. Cover the pan, reduce the heat to low, and simmer 15 to 20 minutes, or until the potatoes are tender when pierced with a knife.

2 Meanwhile, bring a small saucepan of water to a boil. Blanch the green beans 2 to 3 minutes, cool under cold water, and set aside in a colander to drain.

3 In a small bowl, whisk together the vinegar, oil, mustard, chives, salt, and pepper; transfer half of the dressing to a medium-size bowl. When the potatoes are done, drain, cool them slightly, and cut into 1-inch cubes. Add the potatoes to the larger bowl of dressing and toss to coat. Cut the tomatoes into wedges.

4 Divide the romaine among 6 salad plates and arrange the potatoes, tomatoes, green beans, and tuna on top. Pour the remaining dressing over the salads and serve.

Serves 6

PER SERVING
EXCHANGES: 1¾ STARCHES, ¼ FRUIT, ½ VEGETABLE,
4 VERY LEAN MEATS, 1 FAT
NUTRIENTS: 4G FAT/22%, 0.7G SATURATED FAT,
165 CALORIES, 23MG CHOLESTEROL, 306MG SODIUM,
15G CARBOHYDRATE, 17G PROTEIN, 3G DIETARY FIBER

Pasta Primavera Salad with Salmon

½ pound fusilli (spiral pasta)
2 pounds fresh or 4 cups frozen asparagus,
   trimmed and cut into 2-inch pieces
One 10-ounce package frozen peas, thawed
1½ cups julienne cucumber
1 cup julienne zucchini
¼ cup lemon juice
1 tablespoon grated lemon zest
1 tablespoon olive oil
One 7-ounce can salmon, drained and broken
   into chunks
¼ teaspoon salt
¼ teaspoon black pepper

1 Bring 2 large pots of water to a boil.

2 In one pot, cook the pasta according to the package directions, or until al dente.

3 Meanwhile, in the second pot, blanch the asparagus about 3 minutes, or until crisp-tender; drain and cool slightly.

4 Drain the pasta and transfer it to a large bowl. Add the asparagus, peas, cucumber, zucchini, lemon juice, lemon zest, and oil, and toss to combine. Add the salmon, salt, and pepper, and toss gently.

Serves 8

PER SERVING
EXCHANGES: 1¾ STARCHES, 1 VEGETABLE,
¾ MEDIUM FAT MEAT
NUTRIENTS: 4G FAT/18%, 0.7G SATURATED FAT,
206 CALORIES, 8MG CHOLESTEROL, 214MG SODIUM,
31G CARBOHYDRATE, 13G PROTEIN, 3G DIETARY FIBER

Potato-Vegetable Salad with Salmon

½ cup plain lowfat yogurt

2 tablespoons plus 1 teaspoon olive oil

2 tablespoons finely chopped fresh dill,
   or 2 teaspoons dried dill

1 tablespoon Dijon mustard

¼ teaspoon black pepper

1½ pounds small red potatoes, boiled, peeled,
   and quartered

½ pound green beans, cut into 1-inch lengths
   and blanched

1⅓ cups grated zucchini

1 cup grated carrots

1 cup finely shredded red cabbage

¾ cup thinly sliced radishes

½ cup frozen lima beans, blanched

Two 7-ounce cans water-packed salmon

2 shallots, finely chopped

1 tablespoon chopped fresh parsley (optional)

¼ teaspoon salt

1 For the dressing, in a small bowl, stir together the yogurt, oil, dill, mustard, and pepper until well blended; set aside.

2 Place the potatoes, green beans, zucchini, carrots, cabbage, radishes, and lima beans in a large bowl and stir to combine.

3 Drain the salmon and add it to the salad. Add the shallots, parsley (if using), and dressing, and stir gently (the salmon should remain in fairly large chunks). Add the salt, stir again, and serve.

Serves 6

PER SERVING

EXCHANGES: 1¼ STARCHES, 2¼ VEGETABLES,
2 LEAN MEATS
NUTRIENTS: 7G FAT/26%, 1.2G SATURATED FAT,
246 CALORIES, 27MG CHOLESTEROL, 481MG SODIUM,
30G CARBOHYDRATE, 17G PROTEIN, 4G DIETARY FIBER

Bean and Tuna Salad

6 tablespoons lemon juice

1 tablespoon olive oil

2 tablespoons chopped fresh parsley
   (optional)

¼ teaspoon dried rosemary, crushed

¼ teaspoon black pepper

Pinch of salt

2 cups diced carrots

1½ cups coarsely chopped scallions

1 cup diced celery

One 7-ounce can water-packed white tuna

1½ cups canned white beans, rinsed and
   drained

12 large Boston lettuce leaves

1 For the dressing, in a small bowl, combine the lemon juice, oil, parsley (if using), rosemary, pepper, and salt, and whisk until blended.

2 In a large bowl, toss together the carrots, scallions, and celery.

3 Drain the tuna. Add the beans and tuna to the salad, pour the dressing over it, and toss it gently. Let the salad stand at room temperature at least 30 minutes or refrigerate it at least 2 hours.

4 Meanwhile, wash and dry the lettuce. To serve, line 4 plates with lettuce leaves and spoon the tuna salad on top.

Serves 4

PER SERVING

EXCHANGES: ¾ STARCH, 2½ VEGETABLES,
1½ VERY LEAN MEATS, 1 FAT
NUTRIENTS: 5G FAT/21%, 0.8G SATURATED FAT,
213 CALORIES, 19MG CHOLESTEROL, 469MG SODIUM,
24G CARBOHYDRATE, 19G PROTEIN, 7G DIETARY FIBER

Shrimp and Green Bean Salad

1½ pounds green beans, trimmed and
  cut in half

1 pound medium shrimp in shell

1½ tablespoons white wine vinegar

1 tablespoon vegetable oil

2 tablespoons chopped fresh tarragon,
  or 2 teaspoons dried tarragon

2 tablespoons minced chives or scallion greens

¼ teaspoon salt

¼ teaspoon black pepper

½ cup plain nonfat yogurt

1 tablespoon reduced-fat sour cream

1½ teaspoons Dijon mustard

1 teaspoon tomato paste

1 tablespoon chopped fresh parsley

1 Bring 8 cups of water to a boil in a large saucepan. Add the beans and boil for 6 minutes, or until just tender. Drain the beans and refresh them under cold running water. Pat the beans dry and transfer them to a bowl; set aside.

2 Place 4 cups of water in the saucepan and bring to a simmer. Add the shrimp, cover, and simmer the shrimp until they are opaque, 2 to 3 minutes. Drain the shrimp; when they are cool enough to handle, peel and devein them. Add the shrimp to the beans.

3 In a small bowl, whisk together the vinegar, oil, half of the tarragon, 1 tablespoon of the chives, ⅛ teaspoon of the salt, and ⅛ teaspoon of the pepper. Arrange the shrimp and beans on a serving platter and spoon the vinegar-and-oil marinade over the mixture. Let the dish marinate at room temperature for 30 minutes.

4 Near the end of the marinating time, prepare the dressing: Whisk together the yogurt, sour cream, mustard, and tomato paste. Stir in the parsley and the remaining tarragon, chives, salt, and pepper. Pour the dressing into a small serving bowl and serve it alongside the salad.

Serves 4

PER SERVING

EXCHANGES: 2½ VEGETABLES, ¼ SKIM MILK, 2 VERY LEAN MEATS, 1 FAT
NUTRIENTS: 6G FAT/27%, 1.1G SATURATED FAT, 203 CALORIES, 142MG CHOLESTEROL, 360MG SODIUM, 15G CARBOHYDRATE, 24G PROTEIN, 3G DIETARY FIBER

Fish Chowder

1 tablespoon olive oil

1 cup finely chopped onion

1 garlic clove, peeled and crushed

1½ cups peeled, diced potatoes

3 cups low-sodium chicken stock

Small bay leaf

½ teaspoon salt

1 pound skinless, boneless halibut, cut into
  1-inch chunks

1 cup canned crushed tomatoes

¼ teaspoon dried thyme

¼ teaspoon red pepper flakes

¼ cup chopped fresh parsley (optional)

1 Heat the oil in a large saucepan over medium heat. Add the onion and garlic, and cook 3 to 5 minutes, or until softened.

2 Add the potatoes, stock, bay leaf, and salt, cover the pan, and bring to a simmer. Cook for about 15 minutes, or until the potatoes are tender.

3 Add the halibut, tomatoes, thyme, and red pepper flakes; bring to a slow boil and cook, stirring gently, 1 minute, or until the fish is cooked through. Remove the pan from the heat; remove and discard the bay leaf. Sprinkle the chowder with parsley (if using) and serve.

Serves 4

PER SERVING

EXCHANGES: ½ STARCH, 2 VEGETABLES, 3 VERY LEAN MEATS, 1½ FATS
NUTRIENTS: 8G FAT/29%, 1.5G SATURATED FAT, 248 CALORIES, 36MG CHOLESTEROL, 525MG SODIUM, 18G CARBOHYDRATE, 28G PROTEIN, 2G DIETARY FIBER

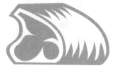

Pepper-Smothered Minute Steak

1 cup rice
½ cup beef stock
2 garlic cloves, minced
1 teaspoon oregano
¼ teaspoon black pepper
3 medium-size bell peppers, cut into thin
    strips
1 small onion, thinly sliced
1 tablespoon olive oil
1 minute steak (about 6 ounces)
1 tablespoon cornstarch

1 In a medium saucepan, bring 2 cups of water to a boil. Add the rice, reduce the heat to low, and simmer for 20 minutes, or until all of the water is absorbed.

2 Meanwhile, in a medium saucepan, bring the beef stock, garlic, oregano, and black pepper to a boil over medium-high heat. Add the bell peppers and onion. Return to a boil, then reduce the heat to low, cover, and simmer 5 minutes.

3 Meanwhile, in a medium nonstick skillet, warm the oil over medium-high heat until hot but not smoking. Add the steak and brown all over, about 3 minutes per side. Remove from the heat and cover loosely.

4 In a small bowl, blend 2 tablespoons of water with the cornstarch. Return the broth and peppers to a boil, stir in the cornstarch mixture, and cook, stirring, until the broth thickens, 1 to 2 minutes.

5 Cut the steak into serving portions; serve over the rice and topped with the peppers. *Serves 4*

PER SERVING
EXCHANGES: 2¼ STARCHES, 1½ VEGETABLES, 1 LEAN MEAT, ½ FAT
NUTRIENTS: 6G FAT/18%, 1.3G SATURATED FAT, 297 CALORIES, 25MG CHOLESTEROL, 234MG SODIUM, 46G CARBOHYDRATE, 14G PROTEIN, 2G DIETARY FIBER

Mexi-Burgers

½ cup canned kidney beans, rinsed and drained
12 ounces extra-lean ground beef
½ cup minced onion
½ cup drained canned diced mild green chilies
½ cup bottled taco sauce
1 garlic clove, minced
1 tablespoon chili powder
1 teaspoon ground cumin
½ teaspoon dried oregano
Four 2-ounce round rolls
1 cup shredded romaine lettuce
2 large plum tomatoes, sliced
¼ cup lowfat sour cream

1 Preheat the broiler. Line a broiler pan with foil.

2 In a medium bowl, mash the kidney beans with a fork. Add the beef, onion, chilies, ¼ cup of the taco sauce, the garlic, chili powder, cumin, and oregano and stir to combine.

3 Divide the mixture into 4 equal portions and shape into patties. Place the patties on the prepared broiler pan and broil 4 inches from the heat for 5 minutes. Turn over and broil for 3 minutes longer, or until the patties are done to your liking.

4 Meanwhile, toast the rolls under the broiler or in a toaster oven.

5 Place one burger on each bun. Dividing evenly, top each burger with the remaining ¼ cup taco sauce, the lettuce, tomatoes, and sour cream. *Serves 4*

PER SERVING
EXCHANGES: 2 STARCHES, 2 VEGETABLES, 2¼ LEAN MEATS, ¾ FAT
NUTRIENTS: 12G FAT/30%, 3.9G SATURATED FAT, 358 CALORIES, 53MG CHOLESTEROL, 782MG SODIUM, 40G CARBOHYDRATE, 26G PROTEIN, 7G DIETARY FIBER

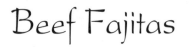

Three-Bean Chili

½ pound extra-lean ground beef
1 cup coarsely chopped onions
1 garlic clove, chopped
1½ cups coarsely chopped green bell pepper
1 cup sliced celery
2 teaspoons chili powder
1 teaspoon ground cumin
½ teaspoon ground oregano
2 cups coarsely chopped fresh tomatoes
¼ cup tomato paste
2 cups no-salt-added crushed tomatoes
1 cup reduced-sodium beef stock
⅔ cup each canned pinto beans, black beans,
    and red kidney beans, rinsed and drained
2 cups hot cooked rice
½ cup coarsely chopped Spanish onion
½ cup shredded cheddar cheese

Heat a large nonstick saucepan over medium heat. Add the beef, onion, and garlic to the pan and sauté until the beef is browned and the onion is translucent. Add 1 cup of the bell pepper and the celery, and continue cooking 5 to 7 minutes, or until the vegetables begin to soften. Add the chili powder, cumin, and oregano, and sauté another minute. Add the fresh tomatoes, tomato paste, crushed tomatoes, the stock, and the drained beans, reduce the heat to medium-low and simmer, partially covered, 30 minutes.

Divide the chili among 4 bowls and top each serving with ½ cup of rice. Sprinkle each serving with the remaining ½ cup of bell pepper, the Spanish onion, and the cheddar cheese.

Serves 4

PER SERVING
EXCHANGES: 3 STARCHES, 4¼ VEGETABLES,
1½ MEDIUM FAT MEATS, 1 FAT
NUTRIENTS: 13G FAT/24%, 5.5G SATURATED FAT,
486 CALORIES, 50MG CHOLESTEROL, 717MG SODIUM,
67G CARBOHYDRATE, 29G PROTEIN, 10G DIETARY FIBER

Beef Fajitas

3 tablespoons cider vinegar
1 tablespoon vegetable oil
3 garlic cloves, minced
2 tablespoons chili powder
1 tablespoon ground cumin
¼ teaspoon red pepper flakes
1 pound lean flank steak
1 large onion
1 large red bell pepper
8 large Boston or Bibb lettuce leaves
¼ cup plain nonfat yogurt

1 In a shallow pan or bowl large enough to hold the steak, combine the vinegar, oil, garlic, chili powder, cumin, and red pepper flakes. Add the flank steak to the marinade and turn to coat completely. Set aside.

2 Preheat the broiler. Line a broiler pan with foil.

3 Halve the onion lengthwise, then cut crosswise into thin half-rings. Cut the bell pepper into thin strips.

4 Place the steak on the broiler pan, reserving the marinade. Broil the meat 4 inches from the heat for 7 minutes. Turn the steak over and broil another 7 minutes, or until medium-rare. Set the steak aside about 5 minutes before slicing; reserve the pan juices.

5 Meanwhile, scrape the reserved marinade into a medium skillet and warm over medium heat until bubbly. Add the onion and bell pepper, and sauté 2 minutes. Reduce the heat to low, cover, and cook 6 minutes, or until the vegetables are crisp-tender. Remove from the heat; when the steak is done, add the pan juices from the steak to the onion mixture.

6 Thinly slice the steak across the grain. Dividing evenly, place the steak strips and onion-pepper mixture on the lettuce leaves. Top with a dollop of yogurt.

Serves 6

PER SERVING
EXCHANGES: 1½ STARCHES, 1½ VEGETABLES,
1½ LEAN MEATS, ¾ FAT
NUTRIENTS: 8G FAT/29%, 2.1G SATURATED FAT,
248 CALORIES, 26MG CHOLESTEROL, 242MG SODIUM,
29G CARBOHYDRATE, 16G PROTEIN, 3G DIETARY FIBER

Beef Enchiladas

1 tablespoon olive oil

2 cups finely chopped onion

1⅓ cups finely chopped green bell pepper

2 cups long-grain white rice

¼ teaspoon salt

2 teaspoons chili powder

½ teaspoon ground cumin

1 cup canned whole tomatoes,
 with their liquid

Eight 6-inch corn tortillas

1 pound lean beef strip steak, well trimmed

2 cups shredded lettuce

2 medium-size fresh tomatoes, diced

½ cup fresh or frozen corn kernels

1 medium-size avocado, peeled and thinly
 sliced

½ cup bottled salsa

1 Heat the oil in a large saucepan over medium-low heat. Add 1 cup of the onions and ⅔ cup of the bell pepper and sauté 4 minutes, or until the vegetables are soft.

2 Add the rice, salt, and half of the chili powder and cumin, and cook, stirring constantly, 1 minute. Add 4 cups of water and the canned tomatoes with their liquid and bring to a boil. Reduce the heat to low and simmer, covered, 20 minutes.

3 Meanwhile, preheat the broiler.

4 Wrap the tortillas tightly in foil and place them on the lower rack of the oven to warm.

5 In a small bowl, combine the remaining chili powder and cumin.

6 Cut the steak in half lengthwise and sprinkle it on all sides with the chili-powder mixture. Place the steak on a broiler pan and broil it 5 inches from the heat for 3 minutes, then turn the steak and broil it another 2 minutes, or until the juices run pink when the meat is pierced. Turn off the broiler, leaving the tortillas in the oven. Slice the steak into 24 thin strips.

7 When the rice is cooked, in a large bowl, toss together the remaining onions and peppers, the lettuce, fresh tomatoes, and corn.

8 Unwrap the tortillas and lay each one on a plate. Spread ¼ cup of rice on each tortilla and top with 3 strips of steak. Divide the vegetable mixture among the tortillas, garnish with avocado slices, and drizzle 1 tablespoon of salsa over each enchilada. Serve the remaining rice on the side. *Serves 8*

PER SERVING

EXCHANGES: 3½ STARCHES, 2 VEGETABLES, 1½ LEAN MEATS, 1¼ FATS
NUTRIENTS: 11G FAT/24%, 2.6G SATURATED FAT, 418 CALORIES, 32MG CHOLESTEROL, 364MG SODIUM, 61G CARBOHYDRATE, 19G PROTEIN, 4G DIETARY FIBER

MEAT BASICS

TO SOME EXTENT, YOU CAN TELL WHICH CUTS OF BEEF, VEAL, LAMB, AND PORK ARE LEAN JUST BY LOOKING AT THEM. FATTY MEAT HAS WHITE STREAKS OR FLECKS OF FAT RUNNING THROUGH THE LEAN RED MUSCLE. EXTERNAL FAT IS TRIMMED QUITE CLOSE ON RETAIL CUTS OF MEAT, BUT YOU CAN FURTHER TRIM OFF ANY REMAINING EXTERNAL FAT BEFORE COOKING THE MEAT.

Marinated Flank Steak with Pilaf

2 teaspoons vegetable oil

1 teaspoon lemon juice

1 teaspoon reduced-sodium soy sauce

1 teaspoon minced garlic

5 ounces lean flank steak

1 cup low-sodium chicken stock

1⅓ cups white rice

2 cups broccoli florets

8 canned water chestnuts, drained and sliced

⅓ cup sliced scallions

2 teaspoons butter or margarine

¼ teaspoon salt

Black pepper

1   In a shallow nonreactive bowl, stir together the oil, lemon juice, soy sauce, and garlic. Add the steak, cover, and marinate in the refrigerator at least 2 hours.

2   About 30 minutes before serving, bring the stock and 1⅔ cups of water to a boil in a medium-size saucepan over medium-high heat. Stir in the rice, cover the pan, reduce the heat to low, and simmer for 20 minutes, or until the rice is tender and the water is completely absorbed.

3   Meanwhile, steam the broccoli 5 minutes, or until tender; set aside. When the rice is done, stir in the broccoli, water chestnuts, scallions, margarine, salt, and pepper to taste; cover the pan and keep warm.

4   Preheat the broiler. Remove the steak from the marinade and place it on a broiler pan. Broil the steak for 4 minutes on each side, brushing it with the marinade as it cooks. (Do not cook the steak beyond the medium-rare stage, or it will become tough.)

5   Cut the steak against the grain into ¼-inch-thick slices and serve it with the rice pilaf.   *Serves 4*

PER SERVING

EXCHANGES: 3 STARCHES, 2¼ VEGETABLES, 1 LEAN MEAT, 1 FAT

NUTRIENTS: 8G FAT/20%, 2.9G SATURATED FAT, 358 CALORIES, 23MG CHOLESTEROL, 277MG SODIUM, 57G CARBOHYDRATE, 15G PROTEIN, 3G DIETARY FIBER

Light Beef Stew

⅓ pound top round steak, well trimmed

1 pound small red potatoes, unpeeled

3 medium carrots

½ pound fresh or 1 cup frozen asparagus

1 bunch scallions (6 to 8)

¼ cup flour

¼ teaspoon pepper

1 tablespoon olive oil

1½ cups beef stock

2 garlic cloves, minced

1½ teaspoons thyme

1 bay leaf

1   Cut the steak, potatoes, and carrots into 1-inch chunks. Trim the asparagus and cut into 1-inch lengths. Coarsely chop the scallions.

2   In a shallow bowl combine the flour and pepper. Dredge the beef lightly in the seasoned flour, reserving the excess.

3   In a large nonstick skillet, warm the oil over medium-high heat until hot but not smoking. Add the beef and cook, stirring frequently, until the meat is browned, about 9 minutes.

4   Meanwhile, add the reserved seasoned flour to the skillet and stir until the flour is no longer visible, about 1 minute. Stir in the beef stock. Add the potatoes, carrots, garlic, thyme, and bay leaf. Bring the stew to a boil, reduce the heat to low, cover, and simmer until the potatoes are tender, about 15 to 20 minutes.

5   Discard the bay leaf. Return the stew to a boil over medium-high heat. Add the asparagus and scallions and cook until the asparagus is just tender, about 5 minutes.   *Serves 6*

PER SERVING

EXCHANGES: 1 STARCH, 2 VEGETABLES, ¾ LEAN MEAT, ¼ FAT

NUTRIENTS: 4G FAT/21%, 0.6G SATURATED FAT, 169 CALORIES, 14MG CHOLESTEROL, 445MG SODIUM, 25G CARBOHYDRATE, 10G PROTEIN, 3G DIETARY FIBER

Sweet Potato Shepherd's Pie

¼ pound extra-lean ground beef
1½ cups diced leeks
1 cup chopped onions
2 garlic cloves, chopped
1 tablespoon plus 1 teaspoon olive oil
2 cups diced celery
2 cups sliced zucchini
1½ cups chopped fresh or canned mushrooms
1 cup frozen corn kernels
½ cup low-sodium chicken stock
2 teaspoons cornstarch
¾ teaspoon dried oregano
1 pound sweet potatoes, cooked
2 tablespoons skim milk
Pinch of ground ginger

1 Heat a large nonstick skillet over medium heat. Add the beef, breaking it up with a spoon, and cook 2 minutes, or until it begins to brown. Add the leeks, onions, and garlic, and cook, stirring, 3 minutes, or until the onions are soft. Add 1 tablespoon of the oil, the celery, zucchini, mushrooms, and corn. Cook, stirring, 2 minutes, or until the celery softens. Add ¼ cup of the stock and bring the mixture to a boil.

2 Meanwhile, in a small bowl, stir together the cornstarch, oregano, and remaining ¼ cup stock. Add this mixture to the skillet and cook, stirring constantly, 1 minute, or until the liquid has thickened; remove the skillet from the heat, cover, and set aside.

3 Preheat the oven to 400°. Peel the sweet potatoes, place them in a large bowl, and mash them with the milk, ginger, and the remaining teaspoon of oil. Scrape the beef mixture into a shallow baking dish and spoon the mashed potatoes in a ring on top. Bake 15 minutes, or until heated through. *Serves 4*

PER SERVING
EXCHANGES: 2¼ STARCHES, 3¾ VEGETABLES, ½ LEAN MEAT, 1½ FATS
NUTRIENTS: 9G FAT/25%, 2G SATURATED FAT, 322 CALORIES, 18MG CHOLESTEROL, 119MG SODIUM, 53G CARBOHYDRATE, 12G PROTEIN, 7G DIETARY FIBER

Split Pea Stew with Spicy Meatballs

¼ pound extra-lean ground beef
1 cup chopped onions
¼ cup dry breadcrumbs
½ teaspoon red pepper flakes
¼ teaspoon dried rosemary, crushed
¼ teaspoon celery salt
2 tablespoons olive oil
1 cup grated carrots
2 cups cooked yellow split peas
2 cups diced cooked parsnips
1½ cups peeled, diced, boiled potatoes
½ teaspoon salt
Black pepper

1 Preheat the oven to 350°. In a medium-size bowl, gently toss together the ground beef, ¼ cup of the onions, the breadcrumbs, red pepper flakes, rosemary, and celery salt. Stir in 2 tablespoons of water. Shape the mixture into 8 meatballs and place them in a baking dish; bake about 15 minutes, or until browned. Set aside.

2 In a large saucepan, heat the oil over medium heat. Stir in the remaining onions and the carrots, and sauté 3 to 5 minutes, or until the vegetables are wilted. Add the peas, parsnips, potatoes, salt, and pepper to taste, then stir in 2 cups of water.

3 Add the meatballs, increase the heat to medium-high, and bring the stew to a boil. Reduce the heat to medium-low, cover, and simmer 20 to 30 minutes, or until the stew is slightly thickened. *Serves 4*

PER SERVING
EXCHANGES: 2½ STARCHES, 4 VEGETABLES, 1½ FATS, ½ VERY LEAN MEAT
NUTRIENTS: 11G FAT/25%, 2.2G SATURATED FAT, 392 CALORIES, 18MG CHOLESTEROL, 415MG SODIUM, 59G CARBOHYDRATE, 18G PROTEIN, 7G DIETARY FIBER

Lamb and Mushroom Stew with Rosemary

2 tablespoons unbleached all-purpose flour
¼ teaspoon each salt and black pepper
½ pound lean stewing lamb, well trimmed,
    cut into 1-inch cubes
1 tablespoon olive oil
One 14-ounce can plum tomatoes,
    with their liquid
¼ pound small fresh mushrooms
1 garlic clove, crushed and peeled
1 bay leaf
¼ teaspoon dried rosemary
2 tablespoons chopped fresh parsley
1 cup long-grain white rice
½ cup frozen peas, thawed

1   Mix the flour, salt, and pepper on a sheet of waxed paper and dredge the lamb cubes in the mixture. Reserve the excess flour.

2   Heat the oil in a large nonstick skillet over medium heat, add the lamb, and sauté 5 to 10 minutes, or until the meat is well browned all over. Add the remaining flour mixture and cook, stirring, 1 minute. Add the tomatoes and their liquid, the mushrooms, garlic, bay leaf, rosemary, and 1 tablespoon of parsley, and bring to a boil. Reduce the heat to medium-low, cover the pan, and simmer the stew 30 minutes.

3   Meanwhile, bring 3 cups of water to a boil in a medium-size saucepan. Stir in the rice, cover the pan, reduce the heat to medium-low, and simmer 20 minutes, or until the rice is tender and the water is completely absorbed.

4   Remove the bay leaf from the stew and stir in the peas. Cover the pan and let stand 5 minutes, then divide the rice among 4 plates, spoon the stew over it, and sprinkle with the remaining parsley.   *Serves 4*

PER SERVING
EXCHANGES: 2½ STARCHES, 2 VEGETABLES, 1½ LEAN MEATS, ¾ FAT
NUTRIENTS: 8G FAT/21%, 2G SATURATED FAT, 338 CALORIES, 37MG CHOLESTEROL, 361MG SODIUM, 49G CARBOHYDRATE, 17G PROTEIN, 3G DIETARY FIBER

Lamb Curry

1 tablespoon plus 1 teaspoon peanut oil
1 cup coarsely chopped onion
1 teaspoon minced garlic
½ teaspoon red pepper flakes
1 teaspoon curry powder
½ pound lean lamb, well trimmed, cut into
    2- x ¼-inch strips
1 cup tomato purée
¾ cup golden raisins
1 tablespoon red wine vinegar
½ teaspoon salt
2 cups cauliflower florets
2 cups green beans, cut into 2-inch pieces
1 cup long-grain white rice
½ cup plain lowfat yogurt

1   In a large heavy saucepan, heat the oil over medium heat. Add the onion, garlic, red pepper flakes, and half of the curry powder, and sauté about 5 minutes, or until the onion is wilted. Stir in the lamb and cook 2 to 3 minutes, or until browned. Stir in 2 cups of water, the tomato purée, raisins, vinegar, salt, and remaining curry powder. Bring to a boil, cover, and simmer 45 minutes, or until the lamb is tender.

2   Meanwhile, bring 1 inch of water to a boil in a medium-size saucepan. Steam the cauliflower and green beans over the boiling water 7 minutes, or until just tender; remove from the pan and set aside.

3   In the same saucepan, bring 2½ cups of water to a boil. Stir in the rice, cover, reduce the heat to low, and cook 20 minutes, or until the water is absorbed.

4   When the lamb is tender, add the cauliflower and beans, cover, and simmer another 5 minutes, or until heated through. Remove the pan from the heat. Stir the yogurt into the curry and serve over the rice.

Serves 4

PER SERVING
EXCHANGES: 2 STARCHES, 1½ FRUITS, 5 VEGETABLES, 1½ LEAN MEATS, 1 FAT
NUTRIENTS: 10G FAT/19%, 2.6G SATURATED FAT, 464 CALORIES, 39MG CHOLESTEROL, 600MG SODIUM, 77G CARBOHYDRATE, 20G PROTEIN, 6G DIETARY FIBER

Citrusy Veal Scallopini

¼ cup fine unseasoned breadcrumbs
¾ teaspoon oregano
¼ teaspoon black pepper
1 egg white
8 veal cutlets (1 pound total)
1 tablespoon olive or other vegetable oil
½ cup chicken stock
1 teaspoon grated lemon zest
2 teaspoons grated orange zest
2 tablespoons lemon juice
1 teaspoon cornstarch
1 garlic clove, minced
2 tablespoons chopped parsley

1 In a shallow bowl, combine the breadcrumbs, oregano, and pepper. In another shallow bowl, beat the egg white. Dip the veal in the beaten egg white, then lightly dredge the veal in the seasoned breadcrumbs.

2 In a large skillet, warm the oil over medium-high heat until hot but not smoking. Add the veal and sauté until golden on both sides, about 3 minutes total. Remove the veal to a plate and cover loosely to keep warm.

3 In a small bowl, stir together the stock, lemon zest, orange zest, lemon juice, cornstarch, garlic, and parsley. Add this mixture to the skillet and stir to combine. Bring the mixture to a boil, return the veal (and any juices that have accumulated on the plate) to the skillet, and cook until heated through, about 1 minute.

4 Top the veal with the pan juices and serve.

Serves 4

PER SERVING

Exchanges: ½ starch, 3½ very lean meats, 1¼ fats
Nutrients: 6g fat/28%, 1g saturated fat, 194 calories, 89mg cholesterol, 272mg sodium, 7g carbohydrate, 26g protein, 0g dietary fiber

Veal Patties in Basil Cream Sauce

1 egg white
4 medium scallions, finely chopped
¼ cup (packed) basil leaves, minced
½ pound ground veal
⅓ cup fine unseasoned breadcrumbs
¾ cup evaporated skim milk
½ teaspoon nutmeg
¼ teaspoon allspice
¼ teaspoon black pepper
1 teaspoon olive oil
1 tablespoon flour
1 cup low-sodium chicken stock

1 In a medium-size bowl, beat the egg white until frothy. Stir in the scallions, half the basil, the veal, breadcrumbs, ¼ cup of the evaporated skim milk, the nutmeg, allspice, and pepper. Form the mixture into 4 patties a scant ½ inch thick.

2 In a large nonstick skillet, warm the oil over medium-high heat until hot but not smoking. Add the patties and cook until browned, 3 to 4 minutes per side. Remove the patties to a plate and cover loosely to keep warm.

3 In a small bowl, combine the remaining ½ cup of evaporated skim milk and the flour, and blend well.

4 Add the chicken stock to the skillet and bring to a boil over medium-high heat, scraping up any browned bits from the bottom of the pan. Stir in the flour-milk mixture and cook, stirring, until the sauce has thickened slightly, about 2 minutes.

5 Stir the remaining basil into the skillet. Return the veal patties (and any juices that have accumulated on the plate) to the skillet and cook until the patties are heated through and well coated with the sauce, 1 to 2 minutes.

Serves 4

PER SERVING

Exchanges: ¾ starch, ½ skim milk, 1¾ very lean meats, 1¼ fats
Nutrients: 6g fat/28%, 2g saturated fat, 194 calories, 48mg cholesterol, 224mg sodium, 17g carbohydrate, 18g protein, 1g dietary fiber

Baked Beans with Bacon

3 strips bacon
1 cup chopped onions
1 cup grated carrots
½ teaspoon dried thyme
1 cup tomato sauce
1 tablespoon tomato paste
1 teaspoon honey
2 cups canned navy beans, rinsed and drained
1 cup fresh breadcrumbs

1 Preheat the oven to 300°. Cook the bacon in a medium-size skillet over medium-low heat about 6 minutes, or until crisp. Reserving the fat in the skillet, remove the bacon. Pat the bacon dry and crumble it; set aside.

2 Pour off all but 4 teaspoons of fat from the skillet; increase the heat to medium and add the onions, carrots, and thyme. Cover the skillet and cook, stirring occasionally, 10 minutes, or until the onion is wilted.

3 Add the bacon, tomato sauce, tomato paste, honey, and ¾ cup of water to the skillet, and stir until well combined. Gently stir in the beans.

4 Sprinkle ¼ cup of the breadcrumbs in the bottom of a 2-quart casserole. Spoon the bean mixture into the casserole and top with the remaining breadcrumbs. Bake about 45 minutes, or until bubbly and browned. Let the dish stand 5 minutes before serving.

Serves 4

PER SERVING
EXCHANGES: 1½ STARCHES, 2¼ VEGETABLES, 1½ FATS
NUTRIENTS: 7G FAT/27%, 2.1G SATURATED FAT, 233 CALORIES, 8MG CHOLESTEROL, 825MG SODIUM, 33G CARBOHYDRATE, 10G PROTEIN, 7G DIETARY FIBER

Braised Pork Chops with Pear

1 small pear
1 small onion
¼ pound green cabbage
2 tablespoons cornstarch
½ teaspoon salt
½ teaspoon black pepper
Four ¼-inch-thick lean center-cut loin pork chops (¾ pound total), well trimmed
1 tablespoon vegetable oil
½ cup frozen apple juice concentrate, thawed
1 tablespoon lemon juice
½ teaspoon caraway seeds, lightly crushed

1 Core and peel the pear and chop it roughly. In a food processor with shredding blade, shred the pear, onion, and cabbage.

2 In a shallow bowl, combine the cornstarch with ¼ teaspoon of the salt and ¼ teaspoon of the pepper. Dredge the pork chops lightly in the seasoned cornstarch, reserving the excess.

3 In a large nonstick skillet, warm the oil over medium-high heat until hot but not smoking. Add the pork chops and cook 5 minutes per side.

4 Slowly add the apple juice concentrate and bring the liquid back to a boil. Reduce the heat to medium-low, cover, and simmer 5 minutes. Remove the pork chops to a plate and cover loosely.

5 Add the shredded pear, onion, and cabbage to the skillet. Increase the heat to medium-high and bring the mixture to a boil.

6 Meanwhile, in a small bowl, stir together the reserved cornstarch mixture and the lemon juice.

7 Add the caraway seeds, the remaining ¼ teaspoon salt and ¼ teaspoon pepper, and the cornstarch mixture, and stir until slightly thickened. Reduce the heat to medium-low, cover, and simmer, stirring occasionally, 5 minutes, or until the cabbage is just tender.

8 Return the pork chops to the pan and cook them 1 to 2 minutes, or until heated through. Serve the pork chops topped with the cabbage and pear.

Serves 4

PER SERVING
EXCHANGES: 1¼ FRUITS, 1½ VEGETABLES, 1½ LEAN MEATS, ½ FAT
NUTRIENTS: 7G FAT/29%, 1.4G SATURATED FAT, 220 CALORIES, 35MG CHOLESTEROL, 188MG SODIUM, 27G CARBOHYDRATE, 13G PROTEIN, 2G DIETARY FIBER

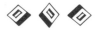

Pork with Sweet-and-Sour Cabbage

Four ¼-inch-thick center-cut lean, well-
trimmed loin pork medallions
(¾ pound total)
2 tablespoons Dijon mustard
1 pound small new potatoes
1 medium-size apple
1 tablespoon olive oil
4 cups shredded red cabbage
2 tablespoons cider vinegar
½ cup unsweetened apple juice
¼ cup chopped fresh parsley (optional)
2 teaspoons butter or margarine
2 tablespoons unbleached all-purpose flour
2 tablespoons sherry

1 Spread the mustard over the pork; wrap it loosely in plastic wrap and refrigerate until needed.

2 Scrub the potatoes, place them in a medium-size saucepan with cold water to cover, and bring to a boil over medium-high heat. Cover the pan, reduce the heat to medium-low, and simmer the potatoes 20 minutes, or until tender.

3 Meanwhile, core and quarter the apple and cut it into ¼-inch-thick slices. Heat 1½ teaspoons of the oil in a medium-size skillet over medium-high heat until hot but not smoking. Add the apple and sauté 3 minutes. Add the cabbage, vinegar, and apple juice, bring to a boil, and cover the skillet. Reduce the heat to medium and cook 5 minutes, then uncover the skillet and increase the heat to medium-high. Cook, stirring constantly, 5 minutes, or until the liquid is almost completely evaporated. Remove the skillet from the heat, stir in 3 tablespoons of the parsley (if using), cover, and set aside.

4 Drain and halve the potatoes, return them to the warm pan, and toss them with the butter and the remaining parsley (if using); cover and set aside.

5 Heat the remaining 1½ teaspoons of oil in a medium-size nonstick skillet over medium-high heat until hot but not smoking. Dredge the pork medallions in the flour and cook them 1 to 2 minutes on each side, or until they are golden brown all over. Add the sherry and 1 tablespoon of water, and cook 1 minute more, or until the pan juices thicken. Divide the pork medallions, the potatoes, and the cabbage mixture among 4 plates and serve. *Serves 4*

PER SERVING
EXCHANGES: 1¼ STARCHES, ½ FRUIT, 2½ VEGETABLES, 2 LEAN MEATS, ¾ FAT
NUTRIENTS: 10G FAT/26%, 3G SATURATED FAT, 344 CALORIES, 59MG CHOLESTEROL, 272 MG SODIUM, 38G CARBOHYDRATE, 23G PROTEIN, 4G DIETARY FIBER

PORK AND VEAL

✓ MODERN BREEDING AND FEEDING METHODS HAVE GREATLY REDUCED THE FAT CONTENT OF PORK, WHICH HAS ABOUT 30 PERCENT LESS FAT THAN IT DID TEN YEARS AGO. SOME CUTS OF PORK, SUCH AS THE TENDERLOIN, ARE COMPARABLE IN FAT CONTENT TO THE LEANER CUTS OF BEEF.

✓ COMPARED CUT FOR CUT, VEAL IS LOWER IN FAT THAN BEEF. VEAL LEG, ONE OF THE LEANEST CUTS, CONTAINS ROUGHLY THE SAME AMOUNT OF FAT AS SKINLESS CHICKEN BREAST. MOST CUTS OF VEAL ARE TOO LEAN FOR BROILING UNLESS YOU TOP THEM WITH SOME VEGETABLES OR A LOWFAT SAUCE TO HELP CONSERVE THEIR JUICES.

Pork Loin with Potatoes and Carrots

⅓ cup frozen pineapple juice concentrate, thawed

3 tablespoons Dijon mustard

1 teaspoon reduced-sodium soy sauce

¼ teaspoon salt

¼ teaspoon black pepper

6 garlic cloves

1 small boneless pork loin (1¾ pounds), trimmed and tied

1 cup chicken stock

1 pound small red potatoes

3 medium-size carrots

2 teaspoons cornstarch

1 Preheat the oven to 425°.

2 In a small bowl, combine the pineapple juice concentrate, mustard, soy sauce, salt, and pepper.

3 Peel the garlic and cut each clove lengthwise into thirds. With a sharp knife, make 18 slits randomly in the pork loin. Tuck a piece of garlic into each slit.

4 Place the pork loin in a small roasting pan and brush the pork with half of the pineapple-mustard mixture. Pour ½ cup of the stock into the bottom of the pan. Roast the pork loin 30 minutes.

5 Meanwhile, quarter the potatoes. Cut the carrots into ½-inch-thick slices. Spray a shallow pan with nonstick cooking spray, place the vegetables in the pan, and roast them until the pork is done.

6 Reduce the oven temperature to 350°. Brush the pork with the remaining pineapple-mustard mixture and continue roasting until it is cooked through and the internal temperature registers 160° on a meat thermometer, about 45 minutes longer.

7 Remove the pork from the roasting pan and let it rest for 5 minutes before slicing. Meanwhile, skim and discard the fat from the pan juices. Stir together the cornstarch and the remaining ½ cup stock.

8 Add the stock mixture to the roasting pan and set over medium-low heat. Stir to incorporate any browned bits clinging to the pan and cook 2 to 3 minutes, or until the sauce is slightly thickened.

9 Slice the pork and serve it with the roasted vegetables and sauce.

Serves 8

PER SERVING

EXCHANGES: ½ STARCH, ½ FRUIT, 1 VEGETABLE, 2¾ LEAN MEATS

NUTRIENTS: 8G FAT/29%, 2.6G SATURATED FAT, 251 CALORIES, 60MG CHOLESTEROL, 406MG SODIUM, 20G CARBOHYDRATE, 23G PROTEIN, 2G DIETARY FIBER

Vegetable-Topped Baked Potatoes

Four 8-ounce baking potatoes
1 medium-size onion, sliced
1 medium-size eggplant, diced
1 medium-size zucchini, diced
1 medium yellow squash, diced
1 small green bell pepper, diced
1 small red bell pepper, diced
One 15-ounce can whole peeled tomatoes,
    with their liquid
1 garlic clove, crushed
½ teaspoon dried oregano
¼ teaspoon red pepper flakes

1   Preheat the oven to 350°.

2   Scrub and dry the potatoes and prick each one a few times with a sharp knife. Bake the potatoes about 1 hour, or until easily pierced with a fork.

3   Meanwhile, in a large nonstick skillet, combine the onion, eggplant, zucchini, yellow squash, bell peppers, tomatoes and their liquid, the garlic, oregano, and red pepper flakes. Sauté over medium-high heat, breaking up the vegetables with a spoon, about 8 minutes, or until the vegetables begin to soften. Cover the skillet, reduce the heat to low, and simmer 20 minutes.

4   Halve the baked potatoes lengthwise without cutting through the bottom skin. Separate the halves and top the potatoes with the vegetable mixture.

Serves 4

PER SERVING
EXCHANGES: 2¼ STARCHES, 4 VEGETABLES
NUTRIENTS: 1G FAT/4%, 0.1G SATURATED FAT,
260 CALORIES, 0MG CHOLESTEROL, 195MG SODIUM,
60G CARBOHYDRATE, 8G PROTEIN, 8G DIETARY FIBER

Vegetable Quesadillas

Two 8-inch flour tortillas
2 fresh plum tomatoes, sliced
½ red bell pepper, finely chopped
½ yellow or red bell pepper, finely chopped
2 scallions, finely chopped
1 large carrot, grated
½ cup reduced-fat cheddar cheese, grated
½ cup plain nonfat yogurt
2 tablespoons bottled salsa
1 cup fresh spinach leaves, torn into
    bite-size pieces

1   Heat a medium-size nonstick skillet over medium heat. Place a tortilla in the skillet and warm it 2 to 3 minutes. Turn the tortilla in the skillet and place half of the tomatoes, bell peppers, scallions, and carrot on one-half of the tortilla. Top the vegetables with half of the cheese, yogurt, salsa, and spinach. Fold the tortilla over the filling and cook another 3 minutes, or until the cheese melts.

2   Transfer the quesadilla to a plate, cover it with foil to keep it warm, and make another quesadilla in the same fashion.

Serves 2

PER SERVING
EXCHANGES: 1¼ STARCHES, 2½ VEGETABLES,
¼ SKIM MILK, 1 MEDIUM FAT MEAT, ½ FAT
NUTRIENTS: 8G FAT/26%, 4G SATURATED FAT,
281 CALORIES, 21MG CHOLESTEROL, 637MG SODIUM,
36G CARBOHYDRATE, 18G PROTEIN, 5G DIETARY FIBER

Veggie Tamale Pie

2 cups frozen lima beans, thawed
1 cup spinach leaves
2 scallions, trimmed and coarsely chopped
2 tablespoons tomato paste
1 garlic clove
1 tablespoon plus 1 teaspoon chili powder
1 cup coarsely chopped green bell pepper
½ cup canned or frozen corn kernels
1½ cups yellow cornmeal
Pinch of salt
¼ cup grated cheddar cheese

1 Place the beans, spinach, scallions, tomato paste, garlic, and 2 teaspoons of the chili powder in a food processor or blender and process until puréed, scraping down the sides of the container with a rubber spatula. Stir in the bell pepper and corn.

2 Preheat the oven to 350°.

3 Spray a heavy-gauge ovenproof skillet (preferably cast iron) with nonstick cooking spray; set aside.

4 In a medium-size saucepan over medium heat, combine the cornmeal, salt, remaining chili powder, and 2½ cups of cold water, and cook, stirring constantly, 2 to 3 minutes, or until the mixture thickens and comes to a boil. Remove the pan from the heat and spread two-thirds of the cornmeal mixture in the prepared skillet. Spoon the lima bean purée over it, top with the remaining cornmeal mixture, and sprinkle the pie with cheese.

5 Bake the tamale pie 30 minutes, or until the cheese is melted and the top is lightly browned. To serve, cut the pie into 6 wedges.

Serves 6

PER SERVING

BLES,

D FAT,

MG SODIUM,

IETARY FIBER

Tortillas Rancheras

1½ cups diced plum tomatoes
1 cup diced yellow bell pepper
1 cup diced red bell pepper
½ cup finely chopped scallions
¼ cup freshly squeezed lime juice
Pinch of grated lime zest
½ teaspoon chili powder
½ teaspoon ground cumin
Pinch of red pepper flakes, or to taste
1½ cups canned black beans,
    rinsed and drained
2 teaspoons vegetable oil
Four 7-inch flour tortillas
3 cups shredded romaine lettuce

1 In a medium-size bowl, stir together the tomatoes, bell peppers, scallions, lime juice, lime zest, chili powder, cumin, and red pepper flakes. Add the black beans and stir to combine; set aside.

2 Heat ½ teaspoon of the oil in a medium-size nonstick skillet over medium-high heat. Place a tortilla in the skillet and cook about 1 minute on each side, or until it is warmed and softened. Repeat with the remaining tortillas and place them on 4 plates. Top each tortilla with shredded romaine and spoon the tomato-bean mixture on top.

Serves 4

PER SERVING
EXCHANGES: 2 STARCHES, 1¼ VEGETABLES, 1 FAT
NUTRIENTS: 5G FAT/20%, 0.7G SATURATED FAT,
221 CALORIES, 0MG CHOLESTEROL, 342MG SODIUM,
36G CARBOHYDRATE, 9G PROTEIN, 7G DIETARY FIBER

Potato and Spinach Casserole

4 baking potatoes (2 pounds)
1½ teaspoons dried rosemary, crushed
½ cup sliced onions
2 cups spinach leaves, chopped

1½ cups skim milk

1 egg

¼ cup grated Parmesan cheese

1 tablespoon dry breadcrumbs

1   Preheat the oven to 350°.

2   Scrub and dry the potatoes and slice them ¼ inch thick. Place half of the slices in a 1½-quart baking dish and sprinkle with half of the rosemary. Top the potatoes with half of the onions and spinach. Repeat the layers.

3   Beat together the milk, egg, and 3 tablespoons of the Parmesan; pour the mixture over the vegetables. Cover the dish with foil and bake 50 minutes.

4   Meanwhile, combine the breadcrumbs with the remaining Parmesan; set aside.

5   Remove the casserole from the oven and top it with the Parmesan mixture. Return the casserole to the oven and bake, uncovered, another 10 minutes.

Serves 4

PER SERVING

EXCHANGES: 2¼ STARCHES, ¼ SKIM MILK,
2 VEGETABLES, ½ MEDIUM FAT MEAT
NUTRIENTS: 3G FAT/10%, 1.5G SATURATED FAT,
263 CALORIES, 59MG CHOLESTEROL, 210MG SODIUM,
47G CARBOHYDRATE, 13G PROTEIN, 5G DIETARY FIBER

Spinach-Cheese Pie

2 cups plain lowfat yogurt

1 pound spinach, trimmed

¾ cup lowfat (1%) cottage cheese

3 tablespoons unbleached all-purpose flour

1 cup chopped scallions

¼ cup chopped fresh parsley (optional)

1 teaspoon dried dill

2 teaspoons grated lemon zest

½ teaspoon white pepper

¼ teaspoon salt

2 tablespoons butter or margarine

8 sheets phyllo dough

1   Place a cheesecloth-lined strainer over a bowl. Spoon the yogurt into the strainer, cover it with plastic wrap, and refrigerate 24 hours, or until the yogurt is the consistency of thick sour cream. You should have about 1 cup of yogurt cheese. Discard the whey.

2   Wash but do not dry the spinach. Place it in a large saucepan over medium-high heat, cover, and cook, stirring occasionally, 1 to 2 minutes, or until the spinach is wilted. Drain in a colander, pressing out as much of the water as possible, then set the spinach aside to cool.

3   Preheat the oven to 375°.

4   In a large bowl stir together the yogurt cheese, cottage cheese, flour, scallions, parsley (if using), dill, lemon zest, pepper, and salt. Squeeze any excess moisture from the spinach. Coarsely chop the spinach and add it to the cheese mixture; set aside.

5   Melt the butter in a small saucepan over medium-low heat; set aside.

6   Unfold the phyllo and cover it with a damp kitchen towel (keep the phyllo covered while you work to keep it from drying out). Place 1 sheet of phyllo in a 9-inch tart pan (preferably with a removable bottom), and brush it lightly with butter. Place another sheet of phyllo in the pan at right angles to the first to form a cross, and brush it with butter. Layer in the remaining phyllo sheets in crisscross fashion to form an even overhang of pastry around the pan, brushing each sheet with butter.

7   Spoon the cheese mixture into the pan and bring the overhanging edges of the phyllo over it to cover it completely. Brush the top with the remaining butter and bake 20 minutes, or until golden brown.

8   Remove the sides of the pan, leaving the pie on the pan bottom, and transfer it to a platter. (If using a regular tart pan, serve directly from the pan.) Cut the pie into quarters and serve.

Serves 4

PER SERVING

EXCHANGES: 1¼ STARCHES, ¾ SKIM MILK, 1 VEGETABLE,
¾ LEAN MEAT, 1½ FATS
NUTRIENTS: 10G FAT/30%, 4.2G SATURATED FAT,
294 CALORIES, 20MG CHOLESTEROL, 654MG SODIUM,
33G CARBOHYDRATE, 17G PROTEIN, 3G DIETARY FIBER

Herbed Potatoes au Gratin

1½ pounds new potatoes
1 tablespoon butter
1 tablespoon unbleached all-purpose flour
¼ cup chopped fresh parsley (optional)
½ teaspoon dried rosemary, crushed
1 teaspoon minced garlic
¼ teaspoon black pepper
1½ cups skim milk
¾ cup sliced onions
2 tablespoons grated Swiss cheese

1 Preheat the oven to 375°.

2 Slice the unpeeled potatoes ¼ inch thick and place them in a bowl of cold water.

3 Melt the butter in a small saucepan over medium-low heat. Stir in the flour, half the parsley (if using), the rosemary, garlic, and pepper. Gradually add the milk, stirring until thick and smooth; set aside.

4 Drain and dry the potatoes; place half of them in a 9-inch-round baking dish. Top with half the onions, then layer in the remaining potatoes and onions. Pour on the sauce, cover the dish with foil, and bake 30 minutes. Stir the potatoes gently and bake another 30 minutes. Stir again, sprinkle the cheese on top, and bake, uncovered, 10 to 15 minutes more, or until the cheese is golden brown. Sprinkle with the remaining parsley (if using) and serve. *Serves 4*

PER SERVING
EXCHANGES: 2 STARCHES, ½ SKIM MILK, ½ VEGETABLE, ¾ FAT
NUTRIENTS: 4G FAT/17%, 2.6G SATURATED FAT, 217 CALORIES, 13MG CHOLESTEROL, 99MG SODIUM, 37G CARBOHYDRATE, 8G PROTEIN, 4G DIETARY FIBER

Stuffed Squash with Cheese

2 medium-size acorn squash (1½ pounds each)
2 tablespoons butter or margarine
1 tablespoon minced garlic
1 cup peeled, diced eggplant
1 cup diced red bell pepper
2 cups cooked brown rice (⅔ cup raw)
¼ cup chopped fresh parsley (optional)
1 tablespoon red wine vinegar
¾ teaspoon dried oregano, crumbled
¼ teaspoon black pepper
Pinch of salt
¾ cup grated part-skim mozzarella

1 Preheat the oven to 375°.

2 Using a large, heavy knife, carefully halve the squash lengthwise. Place the halves cut side down on a foil-lined baking sheet and bake 25 minutes, or until the flesh is barely tender. Leave the oven set at 375°.

3 Let the squash cool slightly, then remove and discard the seeds and stringy membranes. Using a teaspoon, scoop out and reserve the flesh, leaving a ¼-inch-thick shell and being careful not to pierce the skin; set aside the flesh and hollowed-out squash.

4 Melt 1 tablespoon of the butter in a medium-size skillet over medium heat. Add the garlic and sauté 15 seconds, then add the eggplant and sauté 2 to 3 minutes, or until the eggplant begins to soften. Add the bell pepper and continue cooking, stirring occasionally, 2 minutes. Add remaining butter, the reserved squash flesh, rice, parsley (if using), vinegar, oregano, pepper, and salt, and stir to combine.

5 Divide the mixture among the squash shells, top with the mozzarella, and bake 10 to 15 minutes, or until the filling is heated through. *Serves 4*

PER SERVING
EXCHANGES: 2¾ STARCHES, 2 VEGETABLES, ½ MEDIUM FAT MEAT, 1½ FATS
NUTRIENTS: 10G FAT/26%, 5.9G SATURATED FAT, 341 CALORIES, 28MG CHOLESTEROL, 202MG SODIUM, 56G CARBOHYDRATE, 10G PROTEIN, 11G DIETARY FIBER

Black Bean Pot Pie

1½ cups canned black beans, rinsed and
  drained
1 cup tomato sauce
2 tablespoons tomato paste
1 cup chopped onion
¼ teaspoon dried oregano, crumbled
½ teaspoon salt
Black pepper
1 pound all-purpose potatoes, peeled, boiled,
  and mashed
½ cup shredded part-skim mozzarella
2 tablespoons nonfat sour cream
1 tablespoon butter, softened

1   In a medium-size saucepan, stir together the beans, tomato sauce and paste, onion, oregano, ¼ cup of water, ¼ teaspoon of salt, and pepper to taste, and bring to a boil over medium heat. Reduce the heat, cover, and simmer 20 minutes, or until the liquid is thickened and the onions are translucent. Spread the mixture in a shallow 1½-quart casserole and set aside to cool.

2   Preheat the oven to 350°.

3   Place the mashed potatoes in a large bowl. Add the mozzarella, sour cream, butter, the remaining ¼ teaspoon of salt, and pepper to taste, and beat until well blended. Spread the potato mixture evenly over the beans. Score the potato topping with a fork and bake the pie 45 minutes, or until the topping is bubbly and golden.   *Serves 4*

PER SERVING
EXCHANGES: 1¾ STARCHES, 2 VEGETABLES,
½ MEDIUM FAT MEAT, ¾ FAT
NUTRIENTS: 6G FAT/22%, 3.3G SATURATED FAT,
241 CALORIES, 16MG CHOLESTEROL, 1,009MG SODIUM,
37G CARBOHYDRATE, 12G PROTEIN, 7G DIETARY FIBER

Twice-Baked Potatoes

Four 5-ounce baking potatoes
1 tablespoon olive oil
1 cup minced scallions
2 garlic cloves, minced
¾ cup plain nonfat yogurt
¼ teaspoon salt
¼ teaspoon black pepper
1½ ounces grated Parmesan cheese
⅛ teaspoon paprika

1   Preheat the oven to 400°. Prick each potato a few times and bake about 40 minutes, or until they are tender. Preheat the broiler.

2   Meanwhile, in a small skillet over medium-high heat, warm the oil until hot but not smoking. Add the scallions and garlic and cook until the scallions are softened, 2 to 3 minutes. Set aside.

3   When the potatoes are cool enough to handle, halve them lengthwise and scoop the flesh into a bowl, leaving a ¼-inch shell. Mash the potato flesh with a fork or potato masher, then stir in the sautéed scallion mixture, the yogurt, salt, and pepper.

4   Divide the mashed potato mixture evenly among the shells, mounding the stuffing in the center. Sprinkle evenly with the Parmesan and paprika. Broil the potatoes on a baking sheet 4 inches from the heat 2 to 3 minutes, or until the tops are golden.   *Serves 4*

PER SERVING
EXCHANGES: 1¾ STARCHES, ¼ SKIM MILK, ½ VEGETABLE,
¼ HIGH FAT MEAT, 1 FAT
NUTRIENTS: 7G FAT/29%, 2.6G SATURATED FAT,
216 CALORIES, 9MG CHOLE   SODIUM,
30G CARBOHYDRATE, 10G

Sweet Potato Pancakes

⅓ cup unbleached all-purpose flour
¼ cup skim milk
1 egg, beaten
½ teaspoon ground ginger
1 pound sweet potatoes, peeled and grated
    (4 cups)
¼ cup chopped scallions
1 tablespoon plus 1 teaspoon vegetable oil

I In a large bowl beat together the flour, milk, egg, and ginger. Stir in the grated potatoes and scallions.

2 In a large nonstick skillet, heat the oil over medium-high heat until very hot but not smoking. Drop six ¼-cup portions of the potato mixture into the skillet and cook 1 minute. Using a spatula, flatten the mixture into ¼-inch-thick cakes, then reduce the heat to medium and cook 2 to 3 minutes longer.

3 Turn the pancakes and cook another 5 minutes, shaking the pan to keep the pancakes from sticking. Turn the pancakes again and drizzle 2 to 3 table-spoons of water into the pan. Increase the heat to medium-high and cook, pressing the pancakes with the spatula to brown them evenly, 2 minutes longer, or until the pancakes are golden brown all over. Transfer the pancakes to a platter and cover loosely with foil.

4 Repeat with the remaining potato mixture. Divide the pancakes among 6 plates and serve.   *Serves 6*

PER SERVING
EXCHANGES: 1¼ STARCHES, ¾ FAT
NUTRIENTS: 4G FAT/28%, 0.7G SATURATED FAT, 127 CALORIES, 36MG CHOLESTEROL, 24MG SODIUM, 19G CARBOHYDRATE, 3G PROTEIN, 2G DIETARY FIBER

Five-Vegetable Hash Browns

1 pound small red potatoes
½ pound carrots
½ pound parsnips
¼ pound sweet potatoes
¼ pound turnips
1 medium-size onion
2 ounces shallots
2 teaspoons margarine
1 tablespoon olive oil
¼ teaspoon salt
Black pepper

I Cut the red potatoes, carrots, parsnips, sweet potatoes, and turnips into ½-inch-thick slices.

2 Bring ¾ cup of water to a boil in a large nonstick skillet over medium-high heat. Add the vegetables, return the water to a boil, and cover the skillet. Cook 5 to 7 minutes, or until vegetables are crisp-tender, stirring the vegetables several times.

3 Meanwhile, peel and thinly slice the onion and shallots. Transfer the cooked vegetables to a bowl and cover loosely with foil.

4 Wipe the skillet with paper towels. Melt the mar-garine in the skillet over medium heat, then add the onion and shallots, and sauté 2 minutes, or until the onion is soft.

5 Drain and discard any liquid from the bowl and return the vegetables to the skillet, then add the oil and salt. Cook the vegetables, stirring, 10 to 15 min-utes, or until tender and browned. Add pepper to taste. Divide the vegetables among 4 plates and serve.   *Serves 4*

PER SERVING
EXCHANGES: 2 STARCHES, 4 VEGETABLES, 1 FAT
NUTRIENTS: 6G FAT/20%, 0.8G SATURATED FAT, 268 CALORIES, 0MG CHOLESTEROL, 217MG SODIUM, 51G CARBOHYDRATE, 5G PROTEIN, 8G DIETARY FIBER

Potato Pizzas

1 package dry yeast
2⅓ cups unbleached all-purpose flour
1 tablespoon margarine, melted
½ teaspoon plus a pinch of salt
4 firm-ripe plum tomatoes
½ pound small red potatoes
1 medium-size red onion
1 tablespoon cornmeal
1 tablespoon olive oil
1 tablespoon grated Parmesan cheese
1 teaspoon dried oregano, crumbled
¼ teaspoon black pepper

1 Place the yeast in a large bowl; add ⅔ cup of warm water and stir to combine; set aside 3 to 5 minutes. Add ⅓ cup of the flour and stir until smooth, then add the margarine, ½ teaspoon of salt, and the remaining flour, and stir until the mixture forms a cohesive dough. Transfer the dough to a lightly floured board and knead 5 minutes, or until the dough is smooth and elastic. Place the dough in a medium-size bowl, cover it with a damp cloth, and set it aside in a warm place to rise 1 hour, or until doubled in bulk.

2 Meanwhile, wash the potatoes, place them in a small saucepan with cold water to cover, and bring to a boil over medium-high heat. Reduce the heat to medium and simmer, uncovered, 10 to 15 minutes, or until the potatoes are just tender when pierced with a sharp knife. Drain the potatoes and set them aside to cool.

3 When the dough has risen, punch it down and divide it into 4 equal pieces. Wrap each piece in plastic wrap and refrigerate until needed. Peel the onion, then cut the tomatoes, onion, and potatoes into ¼-inch-thick slices; cover them loosely with plastic wrap and set aside.

4 Preheat the oven to 500°.

5 Dust a work surface and a rolling pin with cornmeal. Roll each portion of dough into a ball, flatten it into a disk, then roll it out to a 7-inch circle about ⅛ inch thick. Place the circles of dough on a nonstick baking sheet. Top each pizza crust with onions, then with potato and tomato slices. Drizzle the oil over the pizzas, then sprinkle each one with Parmesan, oregano, pepper, and the remaining pinch of salt.

6 Bake the pizzas 10 minutes, then reduce the oven temperature to 400° and bake 5 to 7 minutes longer, or until the crusts are golden.   *Serves 4*

PER SERVING
EXCHANGES: 4 STARCHES, 3 VEGETABLES, 1½ FATS
NUTRIENTS: 8G FAT/18%, 1.3G SATURATED FAT, 412 CALORIES, 1MG CHOLESTEROL, 378MG SODIUM, 74G CARBOHYDRATE, 11G PROTEIN, 5G DIETARY FIBER

Black Bean and Corn Chili

½ cup coarsely chopped onion
2 garlic cloves, chopped
1 tablespoon safflower oil
1½ cups canned black beans, rinsed and drained
1 cup canned tomatoes, with their liquid
1 tablespoon tomato paste
1 cup frozen corn kernels
1 tablespoon chili powder
1 teaspoon ground cumin
½ cup diced green bell pepper

1 Sauté the onion and garlic in the oil in a medium saucepan over medium heat 1 to 2 minutes, or until the onion is translucent. Add the beans, tomatoes and their liquid, tomato paste, corn, chili powder, and cumin, and stir to combine. Reduce the heat, cover the pan, and simmer 15 to 20 minutes.

2 Add the bell pepper and cook another 5 minutes. Ladle the chili into 4 bowls and serve.   *Serves 4*

PER SERVING
EXCHANGES: 1½ STARCHES, 1½ VEGETABLES, 1 FAT
NUTRIENTS: 5G FAT/27%, 0.4G SATURATED FAT, 169 CALORIES, 0MG CHOLESTEROL, 347MG SODIUM, 27G CARBOHYDRATE, 7G PROTEIN, 6G DIETARY FIBER

Pizza with Mushroom Sauce

1½ cups cornmeal

¼ cup grated Parmesan cheese

2 teaspoons olive oil

¾ pound fresh mushrooms, thinly sliced, or 1½ cups rinsed and drained canned mushrooms

1 medium-size onion, peeled and finely chopped

1 garlic clove, crushed

1 cup canned crushed tomatoes, with their liquid

¼ teaspoon dried oregano, crumbled

¼ teaspoon dried basil, crumbled

⅛ teaspoon red pepper flakes

1 cup shredded Swiss cheese

1 For the crust, bring 3½ cups of water to a boil in a large saucepan.

2 Meanwhile, mix 1 cup of cold water with the cornmeal to make a thick paste. Stir the cornmeal mixture into the boiling water and cook, stirring constantly, 10 to 12 minutes, or until thick and smooth. Remove the pan from the heat, stir in the Parmesan, and mix well.

3 Spread the mixture evenly in a 12-inch nonstick pizza pan or spread it in a 12-inch circle on a large baking sheet, smoothing it with a spatula. Let the crust stand at room temperature at least 1 hour, or until thoroughly cool and dry on the surface.

4 Preheat the oven to 350°.

5 Bake the crust 45 minutes.

6 Meanwhile, for the sauce, heat the oil in a large nonstick skillet and add the mushrooms, onion, and garlic. Cook, stirring, until any liquid evaporates and the mushrooms are lightly browned. Add the tomatoes and their liquid, herbs, and red pepper flakes, and cook over low heat, stirring occasionally, another 5 minutes.

7 Spread the sauce over the crust, top with the Swiss cheese, and bake about 5 minutes, or until bubbly and hot.

Serves 4

PER SERVING

EXCHANGES: 2½ STARCHES, 3¼ VEGETABLES, 1 HIGH FAT MEAT, 1 FAT

NUTRIENTS: 13G FAT/30%, 6.5G SATURATED FAT, 390 CALORIES, 30MG CHOLESTEROL, 271MG SODIUM, 52G CARBOHYDRATE, 17G PROTEIN, 5G DIETARY FIBER

Lentil Pilaf

1 cup yellow or brown lentils

2 tablespoons safflower oil

2 garlic cloves, finely chopped

½ pound fresh tomatoes, coarsely chopped

1 cup coarsely chopped carrots

1 cup coarsely chopped green beans

1 cup coarsely chopped scallions

¾ teaspoon ground cumin

¼ teaspoon salt

1 Place the lentils in a medium-size saucepan with 2 cups of water and bring to a boil over medium-high heat. Cover the pan, reduce the heat to low, and simmer 30 minutes, or until the lentils are just tender; set aside to keep warm.

2 Heat 1 tablespoon of the oil in a medium-size nonstick skillet over medium-high heat. Add the garlic and sauté 30 seconds, or just until fragrant. Add the tomatoes, carrots, green beans, scallions, cumin, and salt, and cook, stirring frequently, 5 minutes, or until the vegetables just begin to color. Add the lentils and any liquid in the saucepan, the remaining oil, and cook, stirring, another 5 minutes, or until the lentils are heated through and the vegetables are crisp-tender.

Serves 4

PER SERVING

EXCHANGES: 2 STARCHES, 1½ VEGETABLES, ¾ VERY LEAN MEAT, 1½ FATS

NUTRIENTS: 8G FAT/27%, 0.7G SATURATED FAT, 266 CALORIES, 0MG CHOLESTEROL, 161MG SODIUM, 37G CARBOHYDRATE, 15G PROTEIN, 8G DIETARY FIBER

Brown Rice and Vegetable Risotto

2 tablespoons plus 1 teaspoon butter
   or margarine
2 cups broccoli florets
1 cup julienne carrots
1 cup parsnips, sliced ⅛ inch thick
1½ cups low-sodium chicken stock
½ teaspoon dried oregano
½ teaspoon black pepper
1½ cups chopped scallions
1 cup brown rice
¼ cup grated Parmesan cheese
¼ cup chopped fresh parsley

1   Melt 1 tablespoon of the butter in a large non-stick skillet over medium-high heat. Add the broccoli, carrots, and parsnips, and cook, stirring, 2 minutes, or until the vegetables are well coated with butter. Add ¼ cup of the stock, ¼ teaspoon of the oregano and ¼ teaspoon of the pepper, cover, and cook 2 minutes more. Stir in the scallions. Remove the pan from the heat, transfer the vegetables to a bowl, and cover it loosely to keep warm.

2   Melt the remaining butter in the skillet over medium-high heat. Add the rice, and sauté 2 minutes. Add ¾ cup of water, the remaining stock, oregano, and pepper. Cover the pan, reduce the heat to medium-low, and simmer 45 minutes, or until the rice is tender and the liquid is almost completely absorbed. Stir in the vegetables, Parmesan, and parsley, and cook, stirring, over medium-high heat 1 minute, or until heated through. Divide the risotto among 4 plates and serve.

Serves 4

PER SERVING

EXCHANGES: 2¼ STARCHES, 3¾ VEGETABLES, 2 FATS
NUTRIENTS: 11G FAT/30%, 5.7G SATURATED FAT,
334 CALORIES, 22MG CHOLESTEROL, 244MG SODIUM,
52G CARBOHYDRATE, 11G PROTEIN, 7G DIETARY FIBER

Roasted Vegetables with Garlic Sauce

2 small new potatoes, or 1 medium-size
   baking potato
1 medium-size sweet potato
1 small acorn squash
1 medium-size pear
½ teaspoon olive oil
2 medium-size turnips, trimmed
2 medium-size parsnips, trimmed
2 medium-size red onions
2 heads of garlic
½ teaspoon salt
¾ cup nonfat sour cream
Black pepper

1   Preheat the oven to 500°.

2   Halve the potatoes lengthwise, quarter the squash, and halve the pear; brush the cut sides lightly with oil. Leave the turnips, parsnips, and onions whole. Peel the outer skin from the garlic heads but do not peel or separate the cloves. Arrange the vegetables and pear in a roasting pan, placing the cut vegetables and pear halves cut side up, and sprinkle with salt. Roast about 30 minutes, or until the vegetables are tender when pierced with a fork. Remove the garlic; cover the pan with foil to keep warm.

3   For the sauce, separate the garlic cloves and squeeze the cloves out of their skins into a bowl; discard the skins. Using a fork, mash the garlic and mix in the sour cream and pepper to taste. Arrange the vegetables and pear on a platter and serve the garlic sauce on the side.

Serves 4

PER SERVING

EXCHANGES: 2 STARCHES, ½ FRUIT,
1 OTHER CARBOHYDRATE, 3½ VEGETABLES, ¼ FAT
NUTRIENTS: 2G FAT/6%, 0.2G SATURATED FAT,
328 CALORIES, 0MG CHOLESTEROL, 375MG SODIUM,
72G CARBOHYDRATE, 10G PROTEIN, 12G DIETARY FIBER

Spiced Lentils and Peas with Rice

¾ cup brown rice

2 tablespoons low-sodium chicken stock

1 cup chopped onion

2 garlic cloves, minced

1¼ cups cooked yellow split peas (½ cup dried)

1¼ cups cooked lentils (½ cup dried)

2 teaspoons ground cumin

¾ teaspoon salt

¼ teaspoon black pepper

One 10-ounce package frozen green peas, thawed

½ cup plain lowfat yogurt

1 Bring 1½ cups of water to a boil in a medium-size saucepan. Stir in the rice, reduce the heat to low, cover, and cook 40 minutes, or until the water is completely absorbed. Remove the pan from the heat and set aside.

2 Combine the stock, onion, and garlic in a large saucepan and cook over medium heat 3 minutes. Add the split peas, lentils, cumin, salt, pepper, and ⅔ cup of water; reduce the heat to low, cover, and cook, stirring occasionally, 10 minutes. Add the green peas and cook another 5 minutes, or until the peas are hot.

3 Divide the rice among 4 plates and spoon the lentil mixture on top. Top each serving with 2 tablespoons of yogurt. *Serves 4*

PER SERVING

EXCHANGES: 4¾ STARCHES, 1 VERY LEAN MEAT, ½ FAT
NUTRIENTS: 3G FAT/7%, 0.6G SATURATED FAT, 388 CALORIES, 2MG CHOLESTEROL, 526MG SODIUM, 72G CARBOHYDRATE, 22G PROTEIN, 9G DIETARY FIBER

Stuffed Mushroom Bake

8 very large mushrooms

1 tablespoon olive oil

5 cups coarsely chopped onions

2 tablespoons vegetable stock or water

3 garlic cloves, minced

½ teaspoon dried thyme

½ teaspoon dried rosemary, crushed

½ teaspoon salt

¼ teaspoon black pepper

1½ cups cooked brown rice (½ cup raw)

2¼ cups diced fresh tomatoes

1 teaspoon dried basil

2 tablespoons grated Parmesan cheese

1 Preheat the oven to 350°.

2 Wash the mushrooms; remove and chop the stems. Heat the oil in a medium-size skillet over medium heat. Add the mushroom caps, hollow side up, and sauté 3 minutes. Transfer the mushroom caps to a plate and set aside.

3 Add to the skillet the chopped mushroom stems, half of the onions, 1 tablespoon of stock, the garlic, thyme, rosemary, ¼ teaspoon of salt, and the pepper. Cook, stirring, 5 minutes, then add the rice and cook 3 minutes more. Transfer the rice mixture to a bowl.

4 Heat the remaining stock in the skillet; add the remaining onions and cook, stirring, for 5 minutes. Add the tomatoes, basil, and remaining salt, and cook, stirring, 5 minutes more.

5 Spoon half of the tomato sauce into the bottom of an 8-inch-square baking pan and spoon ¾ cup of the rice mixture on top. Lay the mushroom caps, hollow side up, on the rice, and spoon the remaining rice mixture over and around them. Pour the remaining tomato sauce over the mushrooms and sprinkle them with Parmesan. Cover the pan tightly with foil and bake 15 minutes, or until heated through. *Serves 4*

PER SERVING
EXCHANGES: 1½ STARCHES, 5 VEGETABLES, 1 FAT
NUTRIENTS: 6G FAT/21%, 1.2G SATURATED FAT,
252 CALORIES, 2MG CHOLESTEROL, 372MG SODIUM,
45G CARBOHYDRATE, 8G PROTEIN, 6G DIETARY FIBER

Vegetable Gumbo

2 tablespoons unbleached all-purpose flour
1 tablespoon vegetable oil
3 cups canned plum tomatoes,
    with their liquid
1 cup coarsely chopped onion
1 cup coarsely chopped green bell pepper
1 cup chopped celery
½ teaspoon dried thyme
1 bay leaf
2 tablespoons chopped fresh parsley
¼ teaspoon hot pepper sauce, or to taste
¼ teaspoon salt
¼ teaspoon black pepper
10 ounces fresh or frozen whole okra, trimmed

1   Stir the flour and oil together in a medium-size saucepan over medium heat for about 2 minutes, or until the flour is browned.

2   Add the tomatoes and their liquid, the onion, bell pepper, celery, thyme, bay leaf, parsley, hot pepper sauce, salt, and black pepper. Reduce the heat to low and simmer, uncovered, 20 minutes.

3   Add the okra and cook another 10 minutes.

4   Remove and discard the bay leaf, then ladle the gumbo into 4 bowls and serve.   *Serves 4*

PER SERVING
EXCHANGES: ½ STARCH, 4 VEGETABLES, 1 FAT
NUTRIENTS: 4G FAT/27%, 0.5G SATURATED FAT,
136 CALORIES, 0MG CHOLESTEROL, 471MG SODIUM,
23G CARBOHYDRATE, 4G PROTEIN, 5G DIETARY FIBER

Chili-Bean Sloppy Joes

½ pound red onions
3 tablespoons butter or margarine
1 garlic clove, chopped
One 14-ounce can plum tomatoes,
    with their liquid
2 cups canned kidney beans, rinsed
    and drained
2 tablespoons tomato paste
1½ teaspoons chili powder
Pinch of salt
Four 2-ounce whole-wheat rolls
⅔ cup shredded romaine lettuce

1   Peel and trim the onions. Cut a 1-inch-thick slice from the center of one onion; wrap and set it aside. Coarsely chop the remaining onions.

2   Heat the butter in a medium-size saucepan over medium heat. Add the chopped onions and garlic and sauté 5 minutes, or until the onions are translucent. Add the tomatoes with their liquid, the beans, tomato paste, chili powder, and salt, and bring the mixture to a boil. Cover the pan, reduce the heat to low, and simmer 20 minutes, stirring occasionally.

3   Ten minutes before serving, preheat the oven to 375°. Split the rolls, wrap them in foil, and heat 10 minutes.

4   Meanwhile, cut the reserved onion into 4 slices. Place the rolls on 4 plates and top them with the bean mixture. Garnish each sandwich with romaine and an onion slice, and serve.   *Serves 4*

PER SERVING
EXCHANGES: 2¾ STARCHES, 2½ VEGETABLES, 2½ FATS
NUTRIENTS: 12G FAT/29%, 6G SATURATED FAT,
367 CALORIES, 23MG CHOLESTEROL, 835MG SODIUM,
53G CARBOHYDRATE, 15G PROTEIN, 12G DIETARY FIBER

South of the Border Sandwiches

1 large tomato, coarsely chopped
¼ cup chopped onion
2 teaspoons balsamic vinegar, or to taste
Four 8-inch flour tortillas
½ medium-size avocado
1 cup canned black beans, rinsed and drained
⅛ teaspoon salt
Black pepper
¾ cup shredded iceberg lettuce
¼ cup plain lowfat yogurt

1 Preheat the oven to 350°.

2 For the salsa, in a small bowl, stir together the tomato, onion, and vinegar; set aside.

3 Wrap the tortillas in foil and heat them in the oven 5 minutes.

4 Meanwhile, peel the avocado half and cut it into thin slices. Using a fork or potato masher, coarsely mash the beans, adding a few spoonfuls of water or stock if they are very dry. Stir in the salt and add pepper to taste.

5 Place each tortilla on a plate. Spread one-half of each tortilla with one-fourth of the beans, then divide the salsa, avocado slices, lettuce, and yogurt among them. Fold the tortillas over the filling and serve.

Serves 4

PER SERVING
EXCHANGES: 2 STARCHES, ½ VEGETABLE, 1½ FATS
NUTRIENTS: 7G FAT/28%, 1.2G SATURATED FAT, 222 CALORIES, 1MG CHOLESTEROL, 384MG SODIUM, 33G CARBOHYDRATE, 8G PROTEIN, 5G DIETARY FIBER

Vegetable-Cheddar Melt

1½ cups shredded spinach
1 cup shredded carrots
⅔ cup coarsely chopped mushrooms
⅓ cup coarsely chopped shallots
¼ cup shredded cheddar cheese
¼ cup plain lowfat yogurt
1 tablespoon Dijon mustard
¼ teaspoon black pepper
4 English muffins

1 Preheat the oven to 375°.

2 In a medium-size bowl, combine the spinach, carrots, mushrooms, shallots, cheese, yogurt, mustard, and pepper, and stir with a wooden spoon until well blended; set aside.

3 Split and toast the muffins, then place them cut side up on a baking sheet. Divide the vegetable mixture evenly among the muffin halves and bake 10 minutes, or until heated through. Divide the muffins among 4 plates and serve.

Serves 4

PER SERVING
EXCHANGES: 1¾ STARCHES, 1 VEGETABLE, ¼ HIGH FAT MEAT, ½ FAT
NUTRIENTS: 4G FAT/17%, 2.2G SATURATED FAT, 212 CALORIES, 10MG CHOLESTEROL, 448MG SODIUM, 34G CARBOHYDRATE, 9G PROTEIN, 3G DIETARY FIBER

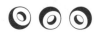

Baked Macaroni and Cheese

¼ cup margarine
1 cup coarsely chopped onion
⅓ cup unbleached all-purpose flour
1 cup skim milk
1 cup chopped fresh tomatoes
¼ cup chopped fresh parsley
1 tablespoon coarse Dijon mustard
1 tablespoon Worcestershire sauce
¼ teaspoon black pepper
10 ounces (2½ cups) elbow macaroni
¼ cup grated cheddar cheese

1 For the sauce, melt the margarine in a medium-size saucepan over medium heat. Add the onion, and cook, stirring, 5 minutes, or until the onion is translucent. Add the flour and stir until well blended. Slowly add the milk, stirring constantly to prevent lumps from forming. Cook the sauce, stirring frequently, another 3 to 5 minutes, or until thickened. Stir in the tomatoes, parsley, mustard, Worcestershire sauce, and pepper, then remove the pan from the heat, cover, and set aside.

2 Preheat the oven to 350°.

3 Meanwhile, bring a large pot of water to a boil. Cook the macaroni 8 minutes, or according to the package directions. Drain the macaroni and transfer it to a 1½-quart baking dish. Add the sauce and stir well. Spread the cheese over the macaroni and bake 10 to 15 minutes, or until the macaroni is heated through and the cheese is melted. Divide the macaroni among 6 plates and serve. *Serves 6*

PER SERVING
EXCHANGES: 3 STARCHES, ½ VEGETABLE, 2 FATS
NUTRIENTS: 10G FAT/28%, 2.4G SATURATED FAT, 324 CALORIES, 6MG CHOLESTEROL, 235MG SODIUM, 47G CARBOHYDRATE, 10G PROTEIN, 2G DIETARY FIBER

Creamy Tuna Mac

1 cup reduced-sodium chicken stock
10 garlic cloves, peeled
¼ cup unbleached all-purpose flour
3 tablespoons plus 1 teaspoon butter
2 cups broccoli florets
1 cup sliced zucchini
1½ cups chopped scallions
½ pound elbow macaroni
One 6⅛-ounce can water-packed tuna
¼ teaspoon black pepper

1 Place the stock and garlic in a medium-size saucepan; add 1 cup of water and bring to a boil over medium-high heat. Cover the pan, reduce the heat to medium-low and simmer for 15 minutes.

2 Meanwhile, knead together the flour and butter until smooth; set aside.

3 Using a slotted spoon, remove the garlic from the pan; set aside. Add the broccoli and zucchini to the pan, cover, and simmer 5 minutes, or until crisp-tender. Stir in the scallions. Reserving the cooking liquid, transfer the vegetables to a serving bowl; set aside.

4 Bring a large pot of water to a boil. Cook the macaroni 10 minutes, or according to package directions.

5 Meanwhile, purée the garlic cloves in a blender.

6 Bring the reserved cooking liquid in the saucepan to a boil over medium-high heat. Whisk in small pieces of the flour mixture until the sauce is smooth and thick, then stir in the garlic purée.

7 Drain the macaroni. Add the macaroni, sauce, tuna, and pepper to the bowl, and stir. *Serves 4*

PER SERVING
EXCHANGES: 3¼ STARCHES, 1½ VEGETABLES, 1½ LEAN MEATS, 1¼ FATS
NUTRIENTS: 11G FAT/23%, 6.2G SATURATED FAT, 427 CALORIES, 42MG CHOLESTEROL, 403MG SODIUM, 58G CARBOHYDRATE, 24G PROTEIN, 5G DIETARY FIBER

Spinach Lasagna

½ pound fresh mushrooms, sliced, or 1 cup
    rinsed and drained canned mushrooms
2 garlic cloves, crushed
1 cup chopped onion
Two 16-ounce cans tomato purée
1 tablespoon dried basil
2 teaspoons dried oregano
¼ teaspoon salt
¼ teaspoon black pepper
¼ teaspoon red pepper flakes
One 10-ounce package lasagna noodles
Two 10-ounce packages frozen chopped
    spinach, thawed
1 tablespoon olive oil
Pinch of ground nutmeg
2 cups lowfat (1%) cottage cheese
2 tablespoons lowfat (1%) milk
2 ounces part-skim mozzarella, shredded
2 tablespoons grated Parmesan cheese

1 Bring a large saucepan of water to a boil.

2 Meanwhile, combine the mushrooms, garlic, and all but 2 tablespoons of onion in a large nonstick skillet; cover and cook over medium heat, stirring often, about 5 minutes, or until the vegetables soften.

3 Add the tomato purée to the skillet. Stir in the basil, oregano, a pinch of salt, a pinch of black pepper, and the red pepper flakes; partially cover and simmer 30 minutes, stirring occasionally.

4 Cook the lasagna noodles according to the package directions; drain and set aside.

5 Preheat the oven to 350°.

6 Squeeze the excess water from the spinach. Cook the reserved onion in the oil in a nonstick skillet until softened. Add the spinach and cook, stirring, until the liquid evaporates. Add the remaining salt and pepper and the nutmeg, and remove the skillet from the heat.

7 Place the cottage cheese and milk in a blender and blend until smooth; set aside.

8 Spread a little tomato sauce on the bottom of a 9- x 13-inch baking dish. Form a layer using one-third of the noodles, one-third of the tomato sauce, half the cottage cheese, half the spinach, and half the

shredded mozzarella. Repeat with one-third of the noodles and the remaining cottage cheese, mozzarella, and spinach. Top with the remaining noodles, tomato sauce, and the grated Parmesan. Cover loosely with foil and bake 50 to 60 minutes, or until bubbly; remove the foil during the last 10 minutes. Let the lasagna stand 10 minutes before serving.

Serves 6

PER SERVING

EXCHANGES: 2¼ STARCHES, ½ OTHER CARBOHYDRATE, 4 VEGETABLES, 1¾ LEAN MEATS
NUTRIENTS: 7G FAT/16%, 2.3G SATURATED FAT, 393 CALORIES, 10MG CHOLESTEROL, 1,153MG SODIUM, 62G CARBOHYDRATE, 25G PROTEIN, 8G DIETARY FIBER

Turkey Tetrazzini

1 cup low-sodium chicken stock
1½ cups sliced fresh mushrooms, or ½ cup
    rinsed and drained canned mushrooms
1 cup chopped red onion
1 cup frozen corn kernels
⅓ cup skim milk
1 tablespoon sherry
1 tablespoon plus 2 teaspoons cornstarch
½ pound skinless cooked turkey breast,
    cut into cubes
1 cup frozen peas
¼ cup chopped fresh parsley (optional)
½ pound fettuccine
2 tablespoons grated Parmesan cheese

1 Bring the stock to a boil in a medium-size saucepan over medium-high heat. Add the mushrooms, onion, and corn, reduce the heat to medium, and simmer the mixture 8 to 10 minutes, or until the mushrooms are tender.

2 Meanwhile, in a small bowl, stir together the milk, sherry, and cornstarch until well blended.

3 Return the stock to a boil, stir in the cornstarch mixture, and boil 2 minutes, or until the sauce thickens. Add the turkey, peas, and parsley (if using), and remove the pan from the heat; cover and set aside.

4 Bring a large pot of water to a boil. Add the fettuccine and cook 10 minutes, or according to the package directions; drain and transfer to a serving bowl.

5 Stir in the turkey mixture and toss until combined, then sprinkle the pasta with Parmesan.

Serves 6

PER SERVING

EXCHANGES: 2½ STARCHES, ½ VEGETABLE, 1¾ VERY LEAN MEATS, ½ FAT
NUTRIENTS: 3G FAT/10%, 0.9G SATURATED FAT, 282 CALORIES, 69MG CHOLESTEROL, 116MG SODIUM, 42G CARBOHYDRATE, 21G PROTEIN, 3G DIETARY FIBER

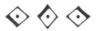

Rotini Salad with Mozzarella and Herbs

10 ounces rotini pasta

2 cups canned crushed tomatoes

½ cup orange juice

2 garlic cloves, minced

3 tablespoons chopped fresh basil, or 1 tablespoon dried basil

1 teaspoon grated orange zest

1 teaspoon ground ginger

½ teaspoon salt

¼ teaspoon black pepper

2 teaspoons olive oil

6 ounces part-skim mozzarella cheese, diced

1 cup thinly sliced celery

1 cup diced orange segments

2 tablespoons chopped fresh parsley (optional)

I Bring a large pot of water to a boil. Cook the rotini in the boiling water until just tender.

2 Meanwhile, in a medium-size saucepan, combine the tomatoes, orange juice, garlic, basil, orange zest, ginger, salt, and pepper. Bring to a boil over high heat and reduce to a simmer. Cover and cook for 5 minutes, or until the garlic is tender and the flavors have blended.

3 Remove the pan from the heat and stir in the oil. Transfer the tomato mixture to a large serving bowl. Cool to room temperature.

4 Drain the pasta, add it to the bowl, and toss to combine. Add the mozzarella, celery, oranges, and parsley (if using) and toss again. Serve chilled or at room temperature.

Serves 4

PER SERVING

EXCHANGES: 3½ STARCHES, ½ FRUIT, 2 VEGETABLES, 1½ MEDIUM FAT MEATS, ½ FAT
NUTRIENTS: 11G FAT/21%, 4.8G SATURATED FAT, 462 CALORIES, 25MG CHOLESTEROL, 699MG SODIUM, 71G CARBOHYDRATE, 22G PROTEIN, 4G DIETARY FIBER

Pasta with Creamy Pesto

2 ounces linguine

½ cup lowfat (1%) cottage cheese

¼ cup fresh basil or cilantro leaves

½ teaspoon salt

2½ teaspoons olive oil

3 garlic cloves, peeled and thinly sliced

¼ teaspoon red pepper flakes, or to taste

I Bring a large pot of water to a boil. Cook the linguine 10 minutes, or according to the package directions; drain and set aside.

2 While the pasta is cooking, place the cottage cheese, basil leaves, and salt in a food processor or blender and process until smooth; set aside.

3 In a small skillet, heat the oil, garlic, and red pepper flakes over very low heat about 5 minutes, or until the garlic is golden. Remove the skillet from the heat, add the drained linguine and the sauce, and toss until well combined.

Serves 2

PER SERVING

EXCHANGES: 1½ STARCHES, 1 LEAN MEAT, ¾ FAT
NUTRIENTS: 7G FAT/30%, 1.2G SATURATED FAT, 209 CALORIES, 2MG CHOLESTEROL, 780MG SODIUM, 26G CARBOHYDRATE, 11G PROTEIN, 1G DIETARY FIBER

Penne with Red Pepper Sauce

3 large red bell peppers, halved and cored
6 ounces penne or other medium pasta
1 tablespoon olive oil
2 medium-size shallots, finely chopped
2 garlic cloves, minced
½ cup white wine
½ cup low-sodium chicken stock
1 medium-size tomato, chopped
2 tablespoons grated Parmesan cheese
1 teaspoon chopped fresh rosemary
½ teaspoon salt
¼ teaspoon black pepper

1 Preheat the broiler.

2 Cut 1 bell pepper into ¼-inch-wide strips; set aside. Broil the other peppers about 5 inches from the heat, turning frequently, until they are charred all over. Place the peppers in a paper bag and let them steam 15 minutes.

3 Meanwhile, bring a large pot of water to a boil. Cook the pasta according to the package directions until al dente; set aside to drain.

4 Chop the roasted bell peppers, place them in a blender, and purée; set aside.

5 Heat the oil in a large nonstick skillet over medium heat. Add the shallots and garlic, and sauté 1 minute. Cover and cook 4 minutes, or until the shallots are soft. Add the wine and stock, bring to a gentle boil, and cook about 3 minutes, or until the liquid is reduced to about ¾ cup. Add the tomato and bell pepper strips and simmer 3 minutes, or until the liquid is reduced to about ½ cup. Add the red pepper purée, half of the cheese, the rosemary, salt, and black pepper, and simmer 1 minute.

6 Toss the sauce with the pasta, then add the remaining cheese and toss again. *Serves 2*

PER SERVING
EXCHANGES: 4 STARCHES, 3 VEGETABLES, ¼ SKIM MILK, 2½ FATS
NUTRIENTS: 12G FAT/21%, 3.1G SATURATED FAT, 517 CALORIES, 7MG CHOLESTEROL, 638MG SODIUM, 80G CARBOHYDRATE, 16G PROTEIN, 5G DIETARY FIBER

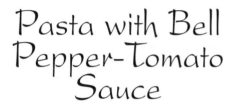

Pasta with Bell Pepper-Tomato Sauce

One 14-ounce can peeled plum tomatoes, with their liquid
1 cup coarsely chopped onion
3 garlic cloves, crushed and peeled
¼ cup chopped fresh basil, or 1 tablespoon dried basil
1 bay leaf
¼ teaspoon black pepper
Pinch of salt
2 large yellow or red bell peppers, slivered
½ pound bow-tie pasta
¼ cup grated Parmesan cheese

1 In a medium-size saucepan, combine the tomatoes and their liquid, the onion, garlic, basil, bay leaf, black pepper, and salt; bring to a boil over medium heat, breaking up the tomatoes with a wooden spoon. Reduce the heat to medium-low and simmer the sauce, uncovered, 15 minutes.

2 Add the bell peppers to the saucepan, cover, and simmer for 15 minutes more.

3 Meanwhile, bring a large pot of water to a boil. Cook the pasta for 10 minutes, or according to the package directions, until al dente.

4 Drain the pasta and divide it among 4 plates. Remove and discard the bay leaf from the sauce. Spoon the sauce over the pasta, then sprinkle 1 tablespoon of Parmesan over each portion. *Serves 4*

PER SERVING

EXCHANGES: 2½ STARCHES, 3 VEGETABLES,
¼ HIGH FAT MEAT
NUTRIENTS: 3G FAT/9%, 1.1G SATURATED FAT,
289 CALORIES, 4MG CHOLESTEROL, 295MG SODIUM,
55G CARBOHYDRATE, 11G PROTEIN, 4G DIETARY FIBER

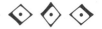

Fettuccine with Vegetables

½ pound green beans
½ pound yellow squash
1 cup lowfat (1%) cottage cheese
⅓ cup skim milk
1 tablespoon butter or margarine
½ pound red onions, sliced
2 garlic cloves, chopped
¾ pound fettuccine
½ teaspoon dried basil
¼ teaspoon white pepper
Pinch of salt
1 tablespoon grated Parmesan cheese

1 Cut the beans into 2-inch lengths. Halve the squash lengthwise and slice it ¼ inch thick; set aside.

2 For the sauce, process the cottage cheese in a blender until smooth. With the machine running, add the milk, and process 5 seconds; set aside.

3 Bring a large pot of water to a boil.

4 Meanwhile, melt the butter in a medium-size skillet over medium heat. Add the onions and garlic, and cook, stirring, 5 minutes.

5 Cook the fettuccine 8 to 10 minutes, or according to the package directions.

6 Meanwhile, add the beans, squash, basil, pepper, and salt to the skillet, and cook, stirring frequently, 10 minutes, or until the vegetables are crisp-tender.

7 Drain the fettuccine and transfer it to a large serving bowl. Add the cheese sauce and vegetables, and toss to combine. Sprinkle the pasta and vegetables with Parmesan and serve.

Serves 4

PER SERVING

EXCHANGES: 4 STARCHES, 2½ VEGETABLES, 1 LEAN MEAT,
1 FAT
NUTRIENTS: 8G FAT/16%, 3.2G SATURATED FAT,
458 CALORIES, 92MG CHOLESTEROL, 354MG SODIUM,
75G CARBOHYDRATE, 23G PROTEIN, 5G DIETARY FIBER

Orzo and Vegetables

2 cups orzo (rice-shaped pasta) or other
    small pasta shape
1 tablespoon vegetable oil
⅓ cup chopped onion
2 medium-size zucchini, cut into 2- x ½-inch
    pieces
1 cup fresh or frozen corn kernels
¼ cup chopped pecans

1 Cook the orzo 8 minutes, or according to the package directions. Turn the orzo into a colander and set aside to drain.

2 Heat the oil in a large skillet. Add the onion and sauté until transparent. Add the zucchini, corn, and ¼ cup water to the skillet; cover and cook the vegetables over medium heat about 5 minutes, or until tender.

3 Add the orzo and pecans to the skillet and cook, stirring, until heated through.

Serves 6

PER SERVING

EXCHANGES: 3¾ STARCHES, ½ VEGETABLE, 1½ FATS
NUTRIENTS: 7G FAT/19%, 0.7G SATURATED FAT,
331 CALORIES, 0MG CHOLESTEROL, 11MG SODIUM,
58G CARBOHYDRATE, 10G PROTEIN, 3G DIETARY FIBER

Pasta with Peppers and Snow Peas

½ pound snow peas
1 green bell pepper
1 yellow or red bell pepper
2 cups broccoli florets
¾ pound linguine
¼ cup reduced-sodium chicken stock
2 tablespoons reduced-sodium soy sauce
2 tablespoons lemon juice
1 tablespoon vegetable oil
2 teaspoons minced fresh ginger
1 garlic clove, minced

1   Bring a large pot of water to a boil.

2   Meanwhile, string and trim the snow peas. Core and coarsely dice the bell peppers; set aside.

3   Blanch the snow peas in the boiling water 30 seconds, or until they turn bright green. Using a slotted spoon and reserving the boiling water, transfer the snow peas to a colander; cool them under cold running water and set them aside to drain. Blanch the broccoli florets 3 minutes, or until crisp-tender; using a slotted spoon, transfer them to a colander, cool, and drain.

4   Return the pot of water to a boil. Cook the linguine in the boiling water 10 minutes, or according to the package directions.

5   Meanwhile, cut the blanched snow peas in half diagonally.

6   For the dressing, combine the stock, soy sauce, lemon juice, oil, ginger, and garlic in a small bowl and stir until blended; set aside.

7   Drain the linguine and transfer it to a large serving bowl. Add the snow peas, bell peppers, broccoli, and dressing and toss to combine.   *Serves 4*

PER SERVING

EXCHANGES: 4 STARCHES, 3 VEGETABLES, 1 FAT
NUTRIENTS: 5G FAT/11%, 0.6G SATURATED FAT, 409 CALORIES, 0MG CHOLESTEROL, 361MG SODIUM, 76G CARBOHYDRATE, 16G PROTEIN, 6G DIETARY FIBER

Spaghetti with Chicken and Bacon

2 tablespoons olive oil
1 ounce Canadian bacon, finely chopped
6 ounces skinless, boneless chicken breast, cut into ½-inch chunks
1 large onion, minced
4 garlic cloves, minced
½ pound fresh mushrooms, thinly sliced, or ⅔ cup rinsed and drained canned mushrooms
2 tablespoons brandy (optional)
2½ cups canned crushed tomatoes
1 teaspoon dried rosemary
½ teaspoon ground black pepper
3 tablespoons chopped fresh parsley (optional)
10 ounces spaghetti

1   Put a large pot of water on to boil. Meanwhile, in a large nonstick skillet, heat 2 teaspoons of the oil over medium heat until hot but not smoking . Add the bacon and cook, stirring frequently, until lightly browned, about 4 minutes. With a slotted spoon, transfer the bacon to a plate.

2   Add 1 tablespoon of the oil to the skillet and heat over medium heat until hot but not smoking. Add the chicken and cook, stirring frequently, until golden brown, about 4 minutes. With a slotted spoon, transfer the chicken to the plate with the bacon.

3   In the same skillet, over medium heat, heat the remaining 1 teaspoon oil until hot but not smoking. Add the onion and garlic and cook, stirring frequently, until the onion begins to brown, about 7 minutes. Add the mushrooms and cook for 2 minutes, or until they begin to soften. Add the brandy (if using), increase the heat to high, and cook until the liquid has evaporated, about 1 minute. Add the tomatoes, rosemary, and pepper and cook until slightly thickened, about 5 minutes. Add the chicken, bacon, and parsley (if using) and simmer until the chicken is cooked through, about 2 minutes longer.

4   Meanwhile, cook the spaghetti in the boiling water until just tender. Drain well. Transfer the chicken mixture to a large bowl, add the spaghetti, and toss to combine. Spoon the chicken and pasta onto 4 plates and serve.   *Serves 4*

PER SERVING
EXCHANGES: 3½ STARCHES, 2½ VEGETABLES, 1½ VERY LEAN MEATS, 2 FATS
NUTRIENTS: 10G FAT/20%, 1.5G SATURATED FAT, 452 CALORIES, 28MG CHOLESTEROL, 382MG SODIUM, 68G CARBOHYDRATE, 24G PROTEIN, 5G DIETARY FIBER

PER SERVING
EXCHANGES: 3¼ STARCHES, 2 FRUITS, 1 MEDIUM FAT MEAT, 1½ FATS
NUTRIENTS: 12G FAT/23%, 5.5G SATURATED FAT, 479 CALORIES, 73MG CHOLESTEROL, 530MG SODIUM, 80G CARBOHYDRATE, 17G PROTEIN, 8G DIETARY FIBER

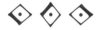

Pasta-Stuffed Peppers

¼ pound fettuccine
2 strips bacon
½ cup finely chopped onion
2 red bell peppers
5 dried figs, diced, or ½ cup raisins
1 tablespoon grated Parmesan cheese
1 ounce goat cheese or lowfat cream cheese
¼ cup low-sodium chicken stock
¼ teaspoon salt
Black pepper

1 Bring a large pot of water to a boil. Cook the fettuccine 8 to 10 minutes, or according to the package directions; drain and set aside.

2 Cook the bacon in a small skillet over medium heat about 7 minutes, or until crisp. Drain the bacon on paper towels, crumble it, and set aside.

3 Drain all but ½ teaspoon of the fat from the skillet. Add the onion and 2 teaspoons of water and cook, covered, over low heat 8 minutes, or until softened; remove the pan from the heat and set aside.

4 Bring another large pot of water to a boil.

5 Meanwhile, cut off and reserve the tops from the bell peppers. Seed the peppers. Blanch the peppers and tops in the boiling water about 10 minutes, or until softened but firm enough to hold their shape. Drain the peppers and tops and set aside to cool.

6 Preheat the oven to 400°.

7 In a large bowl, combine the fettuccine, bacon, onions, figs, Parmesan, cheese, stock, salt, and black pepper to taste, and mix well. Fill each bell pepper with half of the mixture and cover with the tops. Place the peppers in a baking dish and bake about 12 minutes, or until heated through.

Serves 2

Cold Peanut Pasta

¾ pound thin spaghetti
¼ cup smooth peanut butter
1 tablespoon plus 2 teaspoons dark sesame oil
2 tablespoons soy sauce
1 tablespoon Japanese rice vinegar
¼ teaspoon hot pepper sauce
1 cup shredded carrots
1 cup diced green bell pepper
½ cup chopped scallions
2 tablespoons chopped fresh coriander or parsley (optional)

1 Bring a large pot of water to a boil. Cook the pasta 8 minutes, or according to package directions.

2 Drain the pasta in a colander, rinse it under cold running water, and set aside in the colander to drain again.

3 For the sauce, in a small bowl, stir together the peanut butter and oil until blended. Gradually add the soy sauce, vinegar, hot pepper sauce, and 2 tablespoons of water, and stir until smooth.

4 Transfer the pasta to a serving bowl, add the carrots, bell pepper, and scallions, and toss well. Pour on the sauce, sprinkle on the coriander or parsley (if using), and toss until the pasta and vegetables are well coated with sauce.

Serves 6

PER SERVING
EXCHANGES: 2½ STARCHES, 1½ VEGETABLES, ¼ HIGH FAT MEAT, 1½ FATS
NUTRIENTS: 10G FAT/28%, 1.6G SATURATED FAT, 326 CALORIES, 0MG CHOLESTEROL, 411MG SODIUM, 48G CARBOHYDRATE, 11G PROTEIN, 3G DIETARY FIBER

Mexican-Style Pasta with Chicken

4 cups chicken stock

1 garlic clove, minced

1 teaspoon cumin

½ teaspoon chili powder

½ pound skinless, boneless chicken breast

¾ pound thin spaghetti

1 tablespoon vegetable oil

1 can (4 ounces) chopped mild green
    chilies, rinsed and drained

4 plum tomatoes, coarsely chopped

1 large green bell pepper, coarsely chopped

3 scallions, coarsely chopped

¼ teaspoon salt

1 In a medium-size saucepan, bring the stock, garlic, cumin, and chili powder to a boil over medium-high heat.

2 Add the chicken to the boiling stock, reduce the heat to medium-low, cover, and simmer until the chicken is cooked through, about 10 minutes. Remove the chicken to cool slightly.

3 Break the spaghetti into 2-inch pieces.

4 In a large nonstick skillet, warm the oil over medium-high heat until hot but not smoking. Add the spaghetti and cook, stirring until the spaghetti is lightly browned, about 2 minutes.

5 Add the broth mixture, chilies, tomatoes, bell pepper, scallions, and salt, and bring to a boil over medium-high heat. Reduce the heat to low, cover, and simmer, stirring occasionally, until the pasta is cooked, about 7 minutes.

6 Meanwhile, shred the chicken.

7 Stir the shredded chicken into the pasta mixture and serve.

Serves 6

PER SERVING

EXCHANGES: 2¼ STARCHES, 1½ VEGETABLES, 1¼ VERY LEAN MEATS, 1 FAT

NUTRIENTS: 5G FAT/15%, 0.5G SATURATED FAT, 310 CALORIES, 22MG CHOLESTEROL, 826MG SODIUM, 46G CARBOHYDRATE, 18G PROTEIN, 2G DIETARY FIBER

Pasta with Vegetables and Creamy Cheese Sauce

½ pound fresh or 1 cup frozen asparagus

1 medium-size cucumber

1 yellow or red bell pepper

¾ cup reduced-sodium chicken stock

2 teaspoons cornstarch

2 tablespoons butter or margarine

1 cup thinly sliced shallots

¼ cup lowfat (1%) cottage cheese

2 ounces lowfat cream cheese

½ pound medium pasta shells

2 tablespoons chopped fresh basil,
    or 2 teaspoons dried basil

White pepper

1 Trim the asparagus and cucumber. Cut the asparagus into 2-inch lengths. Halve the cucumber lengthwise, then cut it into ¼-inch-thick slices. Seed the bell pepper; cut it into ¾-inch squares. Stir together the stock and cornstarch in a small bowl.

2 Melt the butter in a medium-size skillet over medium heat. Add the shallots and sauté 2 minutes, or until translucent. Add the asparagus, cucumbers, and bell pepper, and cook, stirring, 1 minute, then increase the heat to high. Stir the cornstarch mixture and add it to the skillet. Bring the mixture to a boil, stirring constantly, and cook 2 minutes, or until the asparagus is crisp-tender. Remove the skillet from the heat and carefully pour off the cooking liquid into a small bowl; cover with foil to keep warm. Partially cover the skillet and set aside.

3 Bring a large pot of water to a boil.

4 Meanwhile, place the cheese in a blender. With the machine running, drizzle in the reserved cooking liquid and process 5 to 10 seconds to form a smooth sauce; set aside.

5 Cook the pasta in the boiling water 10 to 12 minutes, or according to the package directions. Drain the pasta thoroughly, transfer it to a large serving bowl, and add the vegetables, sauce, and basil. Add white pepper to taste and toss gently.

Serves 4

PER SERVING

EXCHANGES: 2½ STARCHES, 3 VEGETABLES, ½ VERY LEAN MEAT, 2¼ FATS
NUTRIENTS: 11G FAT/26%, 7G SATURATED FAT, 383 CALORIES, 27MG CHOLESTEROL, 305MG SODIUM, 56G CARBOHYDRATE, 16G PROTEIN, 3G DIETARY FIBER

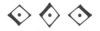

Spaghettini with Artichokes

½ pound fresh mushrooms, or 1 cup rinsed and
    drained canned mushrooms
1 red onion, peeled
2 garlic cloves, peeled
1 cup low-sodium chicken stock
½ cup canned chickpeas, rinsed and drained
3 tablespoons olive oil
½ pound spaghettini or capellini
1½ cups frozen artichoke hearts,
    thawed and drained
1 teaspoon dried oregano, crumbled
Pinch of salt
¼ cup chopped fresh parsley (optional)
¼ teaspoon ground black pepper

1 Wash, trim, and coarsely chop the mushrooms. Coarsely chop the onion and garlic; set aside.

2 Place the stock and chickpeas in a medium-size saucepan and bring to a boil over medium-high heat. Cover the pan, reduce the heat to medium-low, and simmer 15 minutes.

3 Meanwhile, heat 2 tablespoons of oil in a large skillet over medium-high heat. Add the onion and garlic, and cook, stirring occasionally, 10 minutes, or until softened; set aside.

4 Reserving the stock, transfer the chickpeas to a food processor or blender and process until puréed; set aside.

5 Bring a large pot of water to a boil. Cook the spaghettini 8 minutes, or according to the package directions.

6 Meanwhile, return the stock to a boil. Add the mushrooms, artichokes, oregano, and salt, and sim-

mer, stirring occasionally, 5 minutes. Drain the pasta, place it in a serving bowl, and toss it with the remaining oil. Add the chickpea purée, the reserved stock, vegetables, parsley (if using), and pepper and toss again.   *Serves 4*

PER SERVING

EXCHANGES: 3 STARCHES, 2½ VEGETABLES, 2½ FATS
NUTRIENTS: 13G FAT/30%, 1.8G SATURATED FAT, 390 CALORIES, 0MG CHOLESTEROL, 143MG SODIUM, 59G CARBOHYDRATE, 13G PROTEIN, 6G DIETARY FIBER

PASTA SHAPES

THE LIST BELOW OFFERS SOME BASIC GUIDANCE FOR IDENTIFYING DIFFERENT VARIETIES OF PASTA. IF YOU CAN'T FIND A PARTICULAR TYPE OF PASTA CALLED FOR IN A RECIPE, SIMPLY SUBSTITUTE A PASTA OF SIMILAR SIZE OR SHAPE.

CAPELLINI: VERY THIN, ROUND, LONG STRANDS; ALSO CALLED ANGEL HAIR PASTA

CONCHIGLIE: SHELL-SHAPED, IN VARIOUS SIZES; ALSO CALLED PASTA SHELLS

ELBOW MACARONI: SMALL, SHORT, CURVED TUBES

FARFALLE: BUTTERFLY-SHAPED; ALSO CALLED BOW-TIE PASTA

FETTUCCINE: LONG, FLAT STRANDS

LASAGNA: VERY LARGE, FLAT NOODLES

LINGUINE: LONG, THIN, FLAT STRANDS

ORZO: TINY, RICE-SHAPED PASTA

PENNE: TUBES WITH ANGLED ENDS; MAY HAVE SMOOTH OR RIDGED SURFACE

RIGATONI: RIDGED TUBES

ROTINI: SHORT, SPIRAL-SHAPED PASTA; ALSO CALLED PASTA TWISTS OR SPIRAL PASTA

SPAGHETTI: LONG, ROUND STRANDS

SPAGHETTINI: THINNER VERSION OF SPAGHETTI

ZITI: TUBES, LONG OR SHORT

Spaghetti with Tomato-Mushroom Sauce

3 garlic cloves
1 medium-size onion
1 small green bell pepper
½ pound fresh mushrooms, or 1 cup rinsed and
    drained canned mushrooms
3 cans (8 ounces each) tomato sauce
⅓ cup tomato paste
1 bay leaf
1 teaspoon dried oregano
1 teaspoon dried basil
½ teaspoon salt
¼ teaspoon black pepper
¼ teaspoon red pepper flakes
½ pound spaghetti
¼ cup grated Parmesan cheese

1 Bring a large pot of water to a boil.

2 Meanwhile, in a food processor, coarsely chop the garlic, onion, green pepper, and mushrooms.

3 In a medium-size saucepan, combine the chopped vegetables with the tomato sauce, tomato paste, bay leaf, oregano, basil, salt, pepper, and red pepper flakes. Bring to a boil over medium-high heat. Reduce the heat to medium-low, cover, and simmer for 45 minutes.

4 Meanwhile, cook the spaghetti 10 to 12 minutes, or according to the package directions.

5 Remove the bay leaf from the sauce and discard. Serve the spaghetti topped with the sauce. Sprinkle with Parmesan.   *Serves 4*

PER SERVING

EXCHANGES: 2¾ STARCHES, 5 VEGETABLES, ½ FAT
NUTRIENTS: 3G FAT/7%, 1.2G SATURATED FAT,
344 CALORIES, 4MG CHOLESTEROL, 1,575MG SODIUM,
68G CARBOHYDRATE, 14G PROTEIN, 7G DIETARY FIBER

Fettuccine and Carrots with Lemon-Dill Sauce

1 cup lowfat (1%) cottage cheese
¼ cup plain lowfat yogurt
⅓ cup part-skim mozzarella cheese
2 tablespoons grated Parmesan cheese
1½ teaspoons grated lemon zest (optional)
½ cup reduced-sodium chicken stock
3 tablespoons lemon juice
¼ teaspoon white pepper
3 medium carrots, peeled and thinly sliced
3 scallions, coarsely chopped
⅓ cup coarsely chopped fresh dill,
    or 1½ teaspoons dried dill
½ pound fettuccine

1 Bring a large pot of water to a boil.

2 Meanwhile, in a food processor, purée the cottage cheese and yogurt until smooth. Add the mozzarella, Parmesan, and lemon zest (if using), and process to blend.

3 In a medium saucepan, combine the stock, 1 tablespoon of the lemon juice, and the pepper; cover and bring to a boil over medium-high heat. Add the carrots, reduce the heat to low, cover, and simmer until the carrots are crisp-tender, about 5 minutes.

4 Add the scallions and dill to the carrots and continue simmering while the pasta cooks.

5 Add the pasta to the boiling water and cook 8 to 10 minutes, or according to the package directions.

6 Drain the pasta and place it in a serving bowl. Add the broth and carrots, the remaining 2 tablespoons lemon juice, and the cottage cheese mixture. Toss to blend.   *Serves 4*

PER SERVING

EXCHANGES: 3 STARCHES, ½ VEGETABLE,
1½ LEAN MEATS, ¼ FAT
NUTRIENTS: 6G FAT/16%, 2G SATURATED FAT,
333 CALORIES, 64MG CHOLESTEROL, 434MG SODIUM,
50G CARBOHYDRATE, 20G PROTEIN, 4G DIETARY FIBER

Peach and Oatmeal Crisp

2 cups fresh or frozen unsweetened peach slices
¼ cup dried currants or raisins
1 tablespoon honey
¼ teaspoon ground cinnamon
¼ teaspoon vanilla extract
1 cup rolled oats
3 tablespoons unbleached all-purpose flour
1½ teaspoons light brown sugar
1 tablespoon plus 1 teaspoon butter or margarine
1 cup plain lowfat yogurt
1 teaspoon orange juice

1 Preheat the oven to 325°.

2 Reserving 8 thin peach slices for the garnish, in a medium-size bowl combine the remaining peaches, the currants, honey, cinnamon, and vanilla. Spread the mixture evenly in an 8-inch-square pan.

3 For the topping, in a small bowl, stir together the oats, flour, and sugar, then work in the butter with your fingers until the mixture is crumbly. Sprinkle the topping over the peaches and bake 45 minutes, or until the topping is browned. Let the crisp cool for 5 minutes.

4 Meanwhile, stir together the yogurt and orange juice in a small bowl. Divide the peach crisp among 4 plates. Top each serving with ¾ cup of the yogurt mixture and 2 of the reserved peach slices.   *Serves 4*

PER SERVING
EXCHANGES: 1¼ STARCHES, 1¼ FRUITS, ¼ OTHER CARBOHYDRATE, ¼ LOWFAT MILK, 1 FAT
NUTRIENTS: 6G FAT/21%, 3.2G SATURATED FAT, 255 CALORIES, 14MG CHOLESTEROL, 81MG SODIUM, 44G CARBOHYDRATE, 8G PROTEIN, 4G DIETARY FIBER

Nectarine Tart

½ cup rolled oats
1 cup sifted whole-wheat flour
1 teaspoon grated lemon zest
¼ cup reduced-calorie tub margarine
3 to 4 tablespoons ice water
⅓ cup apricot fruit spread
1 tablespoon lemon juice
4 ripe nectarines (about 1½ pounds), cut into ½-inch slices
2 tablespoons toasted sliced almonds

1 Place the oats in a blender and process to the consistency of coarse flour.

2 In a large bowl, combine the oats, flour, and lemon zest. Cut in the margarine until mixture resembles a coarse meal. Sprinkle in the ice water 1 tablespoon at a time until the dough just holds together. Form the dough into a ball, flatten slightly, and wrap in waxed paper. Allow the dough to rest 10 to 15 minutes.

3 Meanwhile, preheat the oven to 425°.

4 On a lightly floured board, roll the dough into an 11-inch disk about ⅛ inch thick. Transfer the dough to a 9-inch pie plate and flute the edge. Bake the pastry shell 12 to 15 minutes, or until lightly browned. Cool completely.

5 Meanwhile, strain the apricot spread into a small saucepan. Add the lemon juice and cook, stirring, over low heat until the jam is thinned and warmed. Brush the inside of the pastry shell lightly with the jam, arrange the nectarine slices in an attractive pattern on top, and brush with the remaining jam. Sprinkle the tart with almonds.   *Serves 6*

PER SERVING
EXCHANGES: 1¾ STARCHES, 1 FRUIT, 1¼ FATS
NUTRIENTS: 6G FAT/23%, 0.9G SATURATED FAT, 232 CALORIES, 0MG CHOLESTEROL, 69MG SODIUM, 42G CARBOHYDRATE, 5G PROTEIN, 5G DIETARY FIBER

Strawberry Shortcake

1 pint fresh strawberries, hulled and sliced
1 tablespoon brown sugar
¼ cup lowfat sour cream
1½ teaspoons grated lemon zest
1¼ cups unbleached all-purpose flour
1 teaspoon baking powder
¼ teaspoon baking soda
¼ teaspoon salt
¼ teaspoon cinnamon
2½ tablespoons soft margarine, well chilled
¼ cup plain lowfat yogurt

1 Toss the strawberries with 1½ teaspoons of the brown sugar.

2 In a small bowl, mix together the sour cream, lemon zest, and remaining brown sugar.

3 Preheat the oven to 450°.

4 In a large bowl, stir together all but 1 tablespoon of the flour, the baking powder, baking soda, salt, and cinnamon. Cut in the margarine until the mixture resembles coarse crumbs. Add the yogurt and ¼ cup of cold water, stir briefly, and form the dough into a ball. On a lightly floured surface, knead the dough a few times, then roll it out to a ½-inch thickness.

5 Using a 3½-inch scalloped cutter, cut out 4 biscuits. Place on a baking sheet and bake 12 to 14 minutes, or until golden. Split the biscuits and place the bottom halves on 4 dessert plates. Top each with one-fourth of the strawberries and 1 tablespoon of the cream; cover with the biscuit tops.   *Serves 4*

PER SERVING

EXCHANGES: 2 STARCHES, ½ FRUIT,
¼ OTHER CARBOHYDRATE, 1¾ FATS
NUTRIENTS: 9G FAT/30%, 2.2G SATURATED FAT,
271 CALORIES, 6MG CHOLESTEROL, 458MG SODIUM,
42G CARBOHYDRATE, 6G PROTEIN, 3G DIETARY FIBER

Butternut Squash Cookies

1 cup unbleached all-purpose flour
1 cup rolled oats
1 teaspoon baking soda
¾ teaspoon ground ginger
¼ teaspoon ground allspice
Pinch of salt
¼ cup butter or margarine, softened
⅓ cup packed brown sugar
1 egg
1 cup cooked butternut or other winter
    squash (see page 88)
½ teaspoon vanilla extract
½ cup each diced dried apricots,
    dried currants, and prunes

1 Preheat the oven to 375°.

2 Lightly spray 2 baking sheets with nonstick cooking spray.

3 In a medium-size bowl stir together the flour, oats, baking soda, ginger, allspice, and salt; set aside.

4 In a large bowl, using an electric mixer, cream the butter and sugar until thoroughly blended. Beat in the egg, then gradually beat in the squash and vanilla. Add the dry ingredients and beat 5 to 10 seconds, or just until mixed, then stir in the apricots, currants, and prunes.

5 Drop the dough by rounded teaspoonfuls onto the baking sheets and bake 12 minutes, or until the cookies are golden at the edges. Transfer the cookies to racks to cool and repeat with the remaining dough.

Makes 96 cookies

PER 3 COOKIES

EXCHANGES: ¼ STARCH, ½ FRUIT, ¼ FAT
NUTRIENTS: 2G FAT/29%, 0.9G SATURATED FAT,
61 CALORIES, 9MG CHOLESTEROL, 55MG SODIUM,
11G CARBOHYDRATE, 1G PROTEIN, 1G DIETARY FIBER

Baked Apricot Custard

¾ cup dried apricot halves
¾ cup pitted prunes
2 eggs
⅓ cup honey
⅔ cup unbleached all-purpose flour
1¾ cups skim milk

1 Place the apricots and prunes in a medium-size bowl, add boiling water to cover, and set aside to soak 1 hour.

2 Preheat the oven to 350°.

3 For the custard, in a small bowl, beat together the eggs and honey until smooth. Gradually whisk in the flour, then stir in the milk.

4 Drain the fruit and divide it among six 8-ounce custard cups or ramekins. Divide the custard among the cups and bake 1 hour, or until the custard is set and golden brown around the edges. Serve the custards warm, or cover them, refrigerate until well chilled and serve cold.

Serves 6

PER SERVING

EXCHANGES: ¾ STARCH, 1½ FRUITS, ¼ SKIM MILK, 1 OTHER CARBOHYDRATE, ¾ MEDIUM FAT MEAT
NUTRIENTS: 2G FAT/7%, 0.6G SATURATED FAT, 244 CALORIES, 72MG CHOLESTEROL, 62MG SODIUM, 52G CARBOHYDRATE, 7G PROTEIN, 3G DIETARY FIBER

Fruit Fold-Ups

1 cup unbleached all-purpose flour
2 tablespoons sugar
2 tablespoons butter or margarine, well chilled
½ cup lowfat (1%) cottage cheese
½ cup dark raisins
3 tablespoons coarsely chopped walnuts
¼ teaspoon ground cinnamon
¼ teaspoon vanilla extract
3 tablespoons strawberry fruit spread

1 In a medium-size bowl, stir together all but 1 tablespoon of the flour and the sugar. Using a pastry blender or 2 knives, cut in the butter until the mixture resembles coarse crumbs. Stir in the cottage cheese, then gather the dough into a ball and knead it a few times in the bowl. Loosely cover the bowl of dough and refrigerate 1 hour.

2 Combine the raisins and walnuts on a cutting board and chop them fine; transfer to a small bowl and stir in the cinnamon and vanilla extract.

3 Preheat the oven to 325°.

4 Line a large baking sheet with foil; set aside.

5 Lightly flour a work surface and rolling pin. Divide the dough into 2 equal pieces, roll out each piece into a 5- x 12-inch rectangle. Place one rectangle with a long side toward you. Brush the bottom half with half of the strawberry spread, sprinkle it with half of the raisin mixture, and fold the top half of the dough over to cover the filling. Cut the folded strip crosswise into eight 1½-inch-wide cookies.

6 Place the cookies 2 inches apart on the baking sheet and make 8 more cookies in the same fashion. Bake 30 minutes, or until the cookies are golden brown, then transfer them to racks to cool.

Makes 16 cookies

PER COOKIE

EXCHANGES: ½ STARCH, ¼ FRUIT, ½ FAT
NUTRIENTS: 2G FAT/22%, 1G SATURATED FAT, 83 CALORIES, 4MG CHOLESTEROL, 44MG SODIUM, 14G CARBOHYDRATE, 2G PROTEIN, 1G DIETARY FIBER

Blueberry Cobbler

2 cups fresh or frozen unsweetened
   blueberries, thawed
3 tablespoons maple syrup
½ cup plus 1 tablespoon unbleached
   all-purpose flour
¾ teaspoon baking powder
½ teaspoon ground cinnamon
⅛ teaspoon salt
1 tablespoon plus 1½ teaspoons butter
   or margarine, melted
1 tablespoon skim milk
1 teaspoon grated lemon zest

1 Preheat the oven to 400°.

2 Lightly spray a 9-inch pie plate with nonstick cooking spray; set aside.

3 If using fresh berries, wash, dry, stem, and pick them over. In a small saucepan, combine the blueberries and maple syrup and cook over medium heat, stirring occasionally, 5 minutes, or until the berries are very soft; remove the pan from the heat and set aside.

4 In a medium-size bowl combine ½ cup of flour, the baking powder, cinnamon, and salt, and stir to combine. Stir in the butter, milk, and lemon zest and mix until a soft dough forms. Using the remaining 1 tablespoon of flour, turn the dough onto a lightly floured surface and roll it out with a floured rolling pin to a 9-inch disk about ⅛ inch thick.

5 Stir the berry mixture, pour it into the pie plate, and lay the crust on top. Bake the cobbler 25 minutes. Let it cool 5 minutes before serving, then cut it into quarters and serve warm.   *Serves 4*

PER SERVING
EXCHANGES: ¾ STARCH, ¾ FRUIT,
¾ OTHER CARBOHYDRATE, 1 FAT
NUTRIENTS: 5G FAT/24%, 2.7G SATURATED FAT,
186 CALORIES, 12MG CHOLESTEROL, 213MG SODIUM,
34G CARBOHYDRATE, 2G PROTEIN, 2G DIETARY FIBER

Chocolate Banana Pudding

2 tablespoons sugar
½ ounce semisweet chocolate
2 ripe bananas, peeled
1½ cups plain lowfat yogurt

1 In a small saucepan heat the sugar, chocolate, and 1 tablespoon of water over very low heat, stirring constantly until the chocolate is melted; remove the pan from the heat and set aside.

2 Purée the bananas in a food processor or blender. Add the yogurt and the chocolate mixture, and process 5 to 10 seconds, scraping down the sides of the container with a rubber spatula. Divide the mixture among 4 dessert dishes and refrigerate 2 to 3 hours, or until well chilled.   *Serves 4*

PER SERVING
EXCHANGES: 1 FRUIT, ½ LOWFAT MILK,
½ OTHER CARBOHYDRATE
NUTRIENTS: 3G FAT/18%, 1.6G SATURATED FAT,
147 CALORIES, 5MG CHOLESTEROL, 61MG SODIUM,
28G CARBOHYDRATE, 5G PROTEIN, 1G DIETARY FIBER

Fruit with Lemon Yogurt Sauce

1 cup plain lowfat yogurt
1 tablespoon sugar
2 teaspoons lemon juice
1½ teaspoons grated lemon zest
1 cup diced cantaloupe
1 cup diced honeydew
1 cup diced fresh pineapple
1 cup sliced fresh strawberries
½ cup fresh raspberries
½ cup seedless red grapes
½ cup diced papaya or peaches
2 tablespoons chopped walnuts

1 For the sauce, in a small bowl, stir together the yogurt, sugar, lemon juice, and lemon zest; set aside.

2 Combine all the fruit in a large bowl with half the sauce and toss gently to coat.

3 Divide the fruit mixture between 4 bowls, top each serving with a portion of the remaining sauce, and sprinkle with walnuts.

Serves 4

PER SERVING

EXCHANGES: 1½ FRUITS, ¼ LOWFAT MILK,
¼ OTHER CARBOHYDRATE, ½ FAT
NUTRIENTS: 4G FAT/23%, 0.8G SATURATED FAT,
154 CALORIES, 3MG CHOLESTEROL, 50MG SODIUM,
28G CARBOHYDRATE, 5G PROTEIN, 3G DIETARY FIBER

Fruit Kebabs with Coconut Sauce

½ cup lowfat (1%) cottage cheese
2 tablespoons lowfat vanilla yogurt
2 tablespoons sweetened flaked coconut
2 cups fresh strawberries
6 ounces large seedless grapes (1 cup)
½ large pineapple, halved lengthwise and cut
    into ½-inch-thick triangles

1 For the sauce, combine the cottage cheese, yogurt, and coconut in a food processor or blender, and process until smooth, scraping down the sides of the container with a rubber spatula. Transfer the sauce to a small bowl.

2 Thread the berries, grapes, and pineapple pieces alternately on each of 8 bamboo skewers and serve with the coconut sauce.

Serves 4

PER SERVING

EXCHANGES: 2 FRUITS, ¾ LEAN MEAT
NUTRIENTS: 2G FAT/12%, 1G SATURATED FAT,
146 CALORIES, 1MG CHOLESTEROL, 128MG SODIUM,
30G CARBOHYDRATE, 5G PROTEIN, 4G DIETARY FIBER

Cranberry Poached Pears with Yogurt

2 cups unsweetened cranberry juice
2 teaspoons sugar
2 teaspoons grated lemon zest
1 teaspoon grated orange zest
1 teaspoon vanilla extract
1 cinnamon stick
4 whole cloves
2 large pears, peeled, halved, and cored
1 cup plain lowfat yogurt
2 tablespoons toasted sesame seeds

1 In a medium-size nonreactive saucepan, combine the cranberry juice, sugar, lemon zest, orange zest, vanilla, cinnamon stick, and cloves, and bring to a boil over medium-high heat. Reduce the heat to low and simmer the mixture 5 minutes.

2 Add the pear halves and simmer another 15 minutes, turning occasionally. Remove the pan from the heat; remove and discard the cinnamon stick and the cloves.

3 Transfer the pear halves and poaching liquid to a bowl and set aside to cool to room temperature, basting the pears often with the liquid if they are not completely immersed.

4 Refrigerate the pears at least 30 minutes, or until well chilled. To serve, divide the pear halves among 4 dessert plates, spoon ⅛ cup of yogurt over each serving, and sprinkle with sesame seeds.

Serves 4

PER SERVING

EXCHANGES: 1½ FRUITS, ½ LOWFAT MILK
NUTRIENTS: 3G FAT/19%, 0.9G SATURATED FAT,
156 CALORIES, 3MG CHOLESTEROL, 45MG SODIUM,
28G CARBOHYDRATE, 4G PROTEIN, 3G DIETARY FIBER

Winter Squash Quickbread

1 cup cooked Hubbard or other winter squash,
   or 1 small uncooked squash
6 ounces dried peaches
½ cup apple juice
2 cups unbleached all-purpose flour
½ cup sugar
2 teaspoons baking powder
1 teaspoon ground allspice
½ teaspoon salt
¼ teaspoon baking soda
2 eggs, beaten
1 tablespoon corn oil

1   If using uncooked squash, preheat the oven to 375°.

2   Using a large, heavy knife, carefully halve the squash. Place the halves cut side down on a foil-lined baking sheet and bake 25 to 35 minutes, or until the flesh is tender when pierced with a knife. Reduce the oven temperature to 350°, remove the squash from the oven, and set aside to cool. Meanwhile, coarsely chop the peaches.

3   Bring the apple juice to a boil in a small saucepan over medium heat. Remove the pan from the heat and stir in the peaches; set aside. When the squash is cool enough to handle, remove and discard the seeds and stringy membranes. Measure 1 cup of the cooked flesh into a small bowl and mash it with a fork; set aside. Reserve any remaining squash for another use.

4   Spray a 9- x 5-inch loaf pan with nonstick cooking spray and dust it lightly with flour.

5   In a large bowl, stir together the flour, sugar, baking powder, allspice, salt, and baking soda, and make a well in the center. Add the peaches and apple juice, the eggs, oil, and mashed squash, and mix just until blended.

6   Turn the batter into the prepared pan and bake 1 hour and 15 minutes, or until the loaf pulls away from the sides of the pan. Let the bread cool in the pan 15 minutes, then turn it out onto a rack to cool completely before slicing it.   *Makes 16 slices*

PER SLICE
EXCHANGES: 1 STARCH, ½ FRUIT, ¼ OTHER CARBOHYDRATE, ½ FAT
NUTRIENTS: 2G FAT/14%, 0.3G SATURATED FAT, 132 CALORIES, 27MG CHOLESTEROL, 159MG SODIUM, 27G CARBOHYDRATE, 3G PROTEIN, 1G DIETARY FIBER

Pumpkin-Spice Yeast Bread

½ cup buttermilk
1 tablespoon butter or margarine
2 tablespoons honey
2 teaspoons dry yeast
½ cup cooked or canned pumpkin
½ teaspoon ground allspice
Pinch of salt
½ cup raisins
2½ cups unbleached all-purpose flour

1   Warm the buttermilk and butter in a small saucepan over low heat until the butter melts and the mixture is just tepid. Meanwhile, in a small bowl, stir together the honey, yeast, and 2 tablespoons of warm water (105-115°); set aside 10 minutes.

2   In a large bowl, stir together the pumpkin, allspice, and salt. Stir in the buttermilk and yeast mixtures and the raisins, then gradually add enough flour to form a dough that pulls away from the sides of the bowl.

3   Using the remaining flour, turn the dough out onto a lightly floured board and knead it with floured hands 5 to 10 minutes, or until the dough is smooth and elastic, kneading in more flour if necessary.

4   Spray a large bowl with nonstick cooking spray. Place the dough in the bowl, cover it with a kitchen towel, and let it rise in a draft-free place 30 to 45 minutes, or until doubled in bulk.

5   Spray a baking sheet with nonstick cooking spray. Punch the dough down and shape it into a round loaf. Place the loaf on the baking sheet and let it rise again 20 to 30 minutes, or until doubled in bulk. Meanwhile, preheat the oven to 375°.

6   With a single-edge razor blade or sharp scissors,

cut a cross in the top of the loaf. Bake the bread about 35 minutes, or until the loaf sounds hollow when tapped. Transfer the loaf to a rack to cool before cutting it into slices.   *Makes 8 slices*

PER SLICE

EXCHANGES: 2 STARCHES, ½ FRUIT, ½ OTHER CARBOHYDRATE, ½ FAT
NUTRIENTS: 2G FAT/8%, 1G SATURATED FAT, 212 CALORIES, 4MG CHOLESTEROL, 50MG SODIUM, 43G CARBOHYDRATE, 5G PROTEIN, 2G DIETARY FIBER

Buttermilk Banana Bread

1¼ cups unbleached all-purpose flour

½ teaspoon baking soda

¼ teaspoon salt

1 large egg

⅓ cup honey

2 tablespoons vegetable oil

¼ cup buttermilk

1 cup mashed ripe banana

¼ cup currants or raisins

¼ cup chopped walnuts

1   Preheat the oven to 350°.

2   Spray a 9- x 5-inch loaf pan with nonstick cooking spray; set aside.

3   In a small bowl, combine the flour, baking soda, and salt; set aside.

4   In a large bowl, using an electric mixer, beat together the egg, honey, and oil until smooth. Add half of the flour mixture and beat until smooth. Beat in the buttermilk, then add the remaining flour mixture, blending well after each addition. Add the mashed banana and blend well. Add the currants and walnuts, and stir until combined.

5   Pour the batter into the pan and bake 50 minutes, or until the bread is firm and brown. A toothpick inserted into the loaf should come out almost dry. Turn the bread out onto a rack to cool completely before slicing it.   *Makes 16 slices*

PER SLICE

EXCHANGES: ½ STARCH, ¼ FRUIT, ½ OTHER CARBOHYDRATE, ½ FAT
NUTRIENTS: 3G FAT/25%, 0.5G SATURATED FAT, 110 CALORIES, 13MG CHOLESTEROL, 82MG SODIUM, 19G CARBOHYDRATE, 2G PROTEIN, 1G DIETARY FIBER

Peach Muffins

1¼ cups unbleached all-purpose flour

1 cup ready-to-eat whole-bran cereal

½ cup whole-wheat flour

1 teaspoon baking powder

1 teaspoon baking soda

¼ teaspoon ground cinnamon

1½ cups buttermilk

¼ cup honey

3 tablespoons vegetable oil

2 large eggs, lightly beaten

1½ cups dried peaches, coarsely diced

1   Preheat the oven to 375°.

2   Spray 18 muffin tin cups with nonstick cooking spray or line them with paper liners.

3   In a large bowl, stir together the all-purpose flour, cereal, whole-wheat flour, baking powder, baking soda, and cinnamon, and make a well in the center.

4   In a medium-size bowl, beat together the buttermilk, honey, oil, and eggs. Pour the buttermilk mixture into the dry ingredients, add the peaches, and stir just until combined.

5   Divide the batter among the muffin cups and bake 20 to 25 minutes, or until the muffins are lightly browned.   *Makes 18 muffins*

PER MUFFIN

EXCHANGES: ¾ STARCH, ½ FRUIT, ¼ OTHER CARBOHYDRATE, ¾ FAT
NUTRIENTS: 4G FAT/26%, 0.6G SATURATED FAT, 136 CALORIES, 24MG CHOLESTEROL, 158MG SODIUM, 25G CARBOHYDRATE, 4G PROTEIN, 3G DIETARY FIBER

Blueberry-Oat Bran Muffins

1½ cups fresh or unsweetened frozen
    blueberries, thawed
1 cup buttermilk
¼ cup honey
2 tablespoons vegetable oil
2 egg whites, lightly beaten
1 cup rolled oats
1 cup oat bran
½ cup unbleached all-purpose flour
2 teaspoons baking powder
Pinch of salt

1 Preheat the oven to 375°.

2 Spray 12 muffin tin cups with nonstick cooking spray or line them with paper liners.

3 If using fresh blueberries, wash, dry, and pick them over.

4 In a small bowl, stir together the buttermilk, honey, oil, and egg whites.

5 In a large bowl, stir together the oats, oat bran, flour, baking powder, and salt, and make a well in the center. Pour in the milk mixture and the blueberries, and stir just until combined; do not overmix.

6 Divide the batter among the muffin cups and bake 25 minutes, or until a toothpick inserted into the center of a muffin comes out clean and dry.

Makes 12 muffins

PER MUFFIN
EXCHANGES: 1¼ STARCHES, ¼ FRUIT, ½ FAT
NUTRIENTS: 4G FAT/28%, 0.6G SATURATED FAT,
129 CALORIES, 1MG CHOLESTEROL, 125MG SODIUM,
23G CARBOHYDRATE, 4G PROTEIN, 2G DIETARY FIBER

Orange-Prune Muffins

12 pitted prunes, cut into eighths
¼ cup orange juice
¾ cup buttermilk
1 tablespoon grated orange zest
1¾ cups unbleached all-purpose flour
1 teaspoon baking powder
½ teaspoon baking soda
½ teaspoon salt
¼ cup vegetable oil
2 tablespoons dark brown sugar
1 egg
1 cup cooked oatmeal

1 Preheat the oven to 400°.

2 Spray 12 muffin tin cups with nonstick cooking spray or line them with paper liners.

3 Cook the prunes and orange juice in a small saucepan over medium-low heat 4 minutes. Remove from the heat and stir in the buttermilk and orange zest.

4 In a large bowl, combine the flour, baking powder, baking soda, and salt; make a well in the center.

5 In another medium-size bowl, combine the oil, sugar, and egg, and mix until blended. Add the prunes and oatmeal and mix until blended. Pour the mixture into the well in the dry ingredients and stir until just combined.

6 Divide the batter among the muffin cups and bake 20 minutes, or until the muffins are firm and browned.

Makes 12 muffins

PER MUFFIN
EXCHANGES: 1 STARCH, ½ FRUIT, ¼ OTHER CARBOHYDRATE,
1 FAT
NUTRIENTS: 6G FAT/33%, 0.8G SATURATED FAT,
165 CALORIES, 18MG CHOLESTEROL, 208MG SODIUM,
26G CARBOHYDRATE, 4G PROTEIN, 2G DIETARY FIBER

Zucchini-Raisin Muffins

1½ cups buttermilk
1 cup rolled oats
½ cup ready-to-eat whole-bran cereal
2 tablespoons butter or margarine
2 tablespoons light brown sugar
1 large egg, lightly beaten
1 cup whole-wheat flour
1 teaspoon baking powder
1 teaspoon baking soda
¼ teaspoon salt
¼ teaspoon ground cinnamon
1 cup grated zucchini, squeezed dry
½ cup dark raisins
¼ cup dry-roasted cashews, coarsely chopped

1 Preheat the oven to 400°.

2 Spray 12 muffin tin cups with nonstick cooking spray or line them with paper liners.

3 In a medium-size bowl, stir together the buttermilk, oats, and cereal; set aside 30 minutes.

4 In another medium-size bowl, using an electric mixer, cream together the butter and brown sugar. Beat in the egg, then stir in the flour, baking powder, baking soda, salt, and cinnamon.

5 Add the flour mixture to the oats mixture and stir to combine. Stir in the zucchini, raisins, and cashews, divide the batter among the muffin cups, and bake 35 minutes, or until a toothpick inserted in the center of a muffin comes out clean.

Makes 12 muffins

PER MUFFIN

EXCHANGES: 1¼ STARCHES, ¼ FRUIT, 1 FAT
NUTRIENTS: 5G FAT/30%, 1.8G SATURATED FAT,
149 CALORIES, 24MG CHOLESTEROL, 274MG SODIUM,
23G CARBOHYDRATE, 5G PROTEIN, 3G DIETARY FIBER

Pear Bread Puddings

2 large eggs
2 ripe pears (1 pound total), or 4 juice-packed canned pear halves, drained
2 tablespoons unbleached all-purpose flour
2 tablespoons sugar
1 cup skim milk
1 teaspoon grated lemon zest
1 teaspoon almond extract
4 slices day-old whole-wheat bread, cut into ½-inch cubes

1 Preheat the oven to 375°.

2 Break the eggs into a small bowl and lightly beat them. Peel and core the pears and cut them into ½-inch cubes.

3 In a medium-size bowl, stir together the flour and sugar. Whisking constantly, gradually add the milk. Stir in the eggs, lemon zest, and almond extract.

4 Combine the pears and bread cubes and divide them among four 8-ounce custard cups. Pour the custard over the bread and pears (it will not completely cover them) and stir gently to coat. Bake the puddings 25 to 30 minutes, or until the custard is set and golden brown on top. Serve the bread puddings hot, at room temperature, or chilled. *Serves 4*

PER SERVING

EXCHANGES: 1 STARCH, 1 FRUIT, ¼ SKIM MILK,
½ OTHER CARBOHYDRATE, ½ MEDIUM FAT MEAT, ½ FAT
NUTRIENTS: 4G FAT/16%, 1.1G SATURATED FAT,
232 CALORIES, 107MG CHOLESTEROL, 213MG SODIUM,
41G CARBOHYDRATE, 9G PROTEIN, 5G DIETARY FIBER

Raspberry Freeze with Lemon Sauce

Two 12-ounce packages frozen unsweetened
    raspberries (3 cups), partially thawed
½ cup frozen apple juice concentrate, thawed
½ cup lowfat (2%) milk
¼ cup evaporated skim milk
1½ teaspoons cornstarch
2 teaspoons grated lemon zest
2 large egg whites
2 tablespoons sugar
1 tablespoon lemon juice
2 tablespoons chopped fresh mint, or
    2 teaspoons dried mint

1 In a food processor or blender, process the raspberries and apple juice concentrate until puréed. Pass the purée through a food mill or sieve, then transfer it to a freezer container and freeze it at least 3 hours.

2 Meanwhile, in a medium-size saucepan, stir together the lowfat milk, evaporated milk, and cornstarch until smooth. Add 1 teaspoon of the lemon zest and bring to a boil over medium heat, stirring constantly; remove from the heat and set aside.

3 In a medium-size bowl, whisk together the egg whites, sugar, and lemon juice until frothy, then gradually whisk in the hot milk mixture. Return the mixture to the saucepan, add the mint, and cook over low heat, stirring constantly, 5 minutes, or until the sauce is thickened. Transfer the sauce to a small bowl, cover, and refrigerate until well chilled.

4 To serve, let the raspberry mixture thaw at room temperature 30 minutes, or until soft enough to scoop. Divide the lemon sauce among 6 dessert dishes. Scoop the raspberry freeze into the dishes and garnish with the remaining lemon zest. *Serves 6*

PER SERVING

EXCHANGES: 1¾ FRUITS, ¼ OTHER CARBOHYDRATE,
½ FAT, ¼ VERY LEAN MEAT, ¼ SKIM MILK
NUTRIENTS: 2G FAT/12%, 0.3G SATURATED FAT,
145 CALORIES, 2MG CHOLESTEROL, 47MG SODIUM,
33G CARBOHYDRATE, 4G PROTEIN, 6G DIETARY FIBER

Fresh Citrus Gelatin with Raspberry Sauce

1 tablespoon unflavored gelatin
2 cups orange juice, preferably freshly
    squeezed
1 lime
1 small orange
¾ cup fresh or frozen unsweetened
    raspberries
Orange wedges and fresh raspberries,
    for garnish (optional)

1 Lightly spray four 6-ounce custard cups with nonstick cooking spray. In a small heatproof bowl, sprinkle the gelatin over ¼ cup of the orange juice; set aside.

2 In a saucepan, warm ½ cup of the orange juice over medium heat until hot but not boiling. Add the softened gelatin; stir to dissolve, then set aside.

3 Cut the lime in half crosswise. Cut 4 slices from one half and juice the remaining half.

4 Stir the lime juice and the remaining 1¼ cups orange juice into the gelatin mixture and place it in the refrigerator to cool. Stir the gelatin after 10 minutes to cool it more quickly. Chill the gelatin until it begins to thicken, checking and stirring it about every 2 minutes.

5 Meanwhile, use a sharp knife to peel the orange, removing the pith and the membrane; separate the fruit into sections.

6 Fold the orange sections into the thickened gelatin mixture.

7 Place a slice of lime in the bottom of each custard cup, then divide the gelatin among the 4 cups. Refrigerate 3 hours, or until the gelatin is set.

8 Purée the raspberries in a food processor.

9 Dip each custard cup in hot water for 2 to 5 seconds, or until the gelatin just begins to pull away from the sides of the dish. Invert the cups onto individual dessert dishes and unmold. Spoon the raspberry sauce in a sunburst pattern around the gelatin and garnish the desserts with orange wedges and raspberries, if desired. *Serves 4*

PER SERVING
EXCHANGES: 1½ FRUITS, ¼ VERY LEAN MEAT
NUTRIENTS: 1G FAT/10%, 0G SATURATED FAT,
93 CALORIES, 0MG CHOLESTEROL, 5MG SODIUM,
20G CARBOHYDRATE, 3G PROTEIN, 2G DIETARY FIBER

Oatmeal Scones

1⅓ cups all-purpose flour

1 cup rolled oats

1 tablespoon sugar

1 teaspoon baking soda

Pinch of salt

¼ cup butter or margarine, well chilled

⅔ cup buttermilk

½ cup golden raisins

1 Preheat the oven the 400°.

2 In a food processor, combine 1¼ cups of the flour, the oats, sugar, baking soda, and salt.

3 Cut the butter into small pieces, add it to the dry ingredients, and process, pulsing the machine on and off, 10 seconds, or until the mixture resembles coarse cornmeal. Add the buttermilk and process another 10 seconds, or until the dough forms a ball.

4 Turn the dough out onto a lightly floured board and gently knead in the raisins 2 minutes, or until the dough is smooth.

5 Using a lightly floured rolling pin, roll the dough out into an 8½-inch disk about ½ inch thick. Place the dough on a baking sheet, then, using a sharp knife, lightly score it into 8 wedges. Bake 15 minutes, or until golden. Cool slightly, then cut the scones along the scored lines.

Makes 8 scones

PER SCONE
EXCHANGES: 1½ STARCHES, ½ FRUIT, 1½ FATS
NUTRIENTS: 7G FAT/30%, 3.8G SATURATED FAT,
207 CALORIES, 16MG CHOLESTEROL, 256MG SODIUM,
32G CARBOHYDRATE, 5G PROTEIN, 2G DIETARY FIBER

Oatmeal Banana Bars

1 tablespoon margarine

1 tablespoon brown sugar

1 cup rolled oats

¼ teaspoon ground cinnamon

½ cup whole-wheat flour

½ cup apple juice

½ teaspoon vanilla extract

1 banana, mashed

¼ cup dried currants or raisins

1 Preheat the oven to 350°. Spray an 8-inch-square baking pan with nonstick cooking spray. In a medium-size bowl, beat together the margarine and sugar until creamy. Stir in the oats and cinnamon until combined, then add the flour and stir until combined.

2 Mix the apple juice, vanilla, and ½ cup of warm water in a small bowl, then add this mixture to the dry ingredients and stir well. Stir in the mashed banana and currants.

3 Spread the dough into the prepared baking pan, smoothing the top with a rubber spatula, and bake for about 1 hour, or until the top is golden. Let the cake cool in the pan on a rack. To serve, cut the cake into quarters, then cut each quarter into 3 bars.

Makes 12 bars

PER BAR
EXCHANGES: ¾ STARCH, ¼ FRUIT, ¼ FAT
NUTRIENTS: 2G FAT/23%, 0.2G SATURATED FAT,
79 CALORIES, 0MG CHOLESTEROL, 13MG SODIUM,
15G CARBOHYDRATE, 2G PROTEIN, 2G DIETARY FIBER